Rigid and Contact Endoscopy in Microlaryngeal Surgery

Technique and Atlas of Clinical Cases

To Maurice
hoping that you will
enjoy this book as much
as we have in preparing it

Mario
[illegible]

Lisbon 16/[illegible]

Rigid and Contact Endoscopy in Microlaryngeal Surgery

Technique and Atlas of Clinical Cases

Mário Andrea M.D., Ph.D.
Professor
Director and Chairman
Department of Otolaryngology
Faculty of Medicine of Lisbon
Lisbon, Portugal

Oscar Dias M.D., Ph.D.
Assistant Professor
Department of Otolaryngology
Faculty of Medicine of Lisbon
Lisbon, Portugal

Lippincott - Raven
PUBLISHERS
Philadelphia • New York

Lippincott - Raven Publishers, 227 East Washington Square,
Philadelphia, Pennsylvania 19106-3780

Printed and bound in Hong Kong

Library of Congress Cataloging-in-Publication Data

Andrea, Mário.
Atlas of rigid and contact endoscopy in microlaryngeal surgery / Mário Andrea, Oscar Dias.
p. cm.
Includes bibliographical references and index.
ISBN 0-7817-0328-X
1. Laryngoscopy—Atlases. 2. Larynx—Surgery—Atlases. 3. Microsurgery—Atlases. I. Dias, Oscar II. Title.
[DNLM: 1. Vocal Cords—surgery—atlases. 2. Microsurgery—atlases. 3. Laryngoscopy—atlases. WV 17 A556a 1995]
RF514.A58 1995
617.5'33059—dc20
DNLM/DLC
for Library of Congress

95-14124

The material contained in this volume was submitted as previously unpublished material, except in the instances in which credit has been given to the source from which some of the illustrative material was derived.

Great care has been taken to maintain the accuracy of the information contained in the volume. However, neither Lippincott - Raven Publishers nor the authors can be held responsible for errors or for any consequences arising from the use of the information contained herein.

9 8 7 6 5 4 3 2 1

In memory of my father Fernando, forever in my heart, my spirit, and my mind.

To my mother Maria Octavia, for her love, understanding, and support.

To my wife Jana, for sharing our life together for more than 20 years, and for her love, patience, and continuous support.

To my daughters Monica and Mafalda, with all my love, devotion, and immense pride.

M.A.

To Tulia for her love, support, and understanding she has given me throughout these years.

To Tania, Lisa, and Miguel, who have brought a new meaning to my life and enriched it with their love.

O.D.

Contents

Foreword

This atlas by Mário Andrea and Oscar Dias brings to us their mastery of rigid endoscopy and a new technology that rewrites our understanding of the anatomy and pathology of the larynx and allows a precise microsurgical approach to therapy. This treatise will stimulate and challenge us to conceive new approaches to therapy and surely will stimulate refinements and additions to this exciting technological advance.

The authors meticulously present their innovative approach to rigid endoscopy of the larynx—particularly their innovative and illuminating use of angled telescopes to allow visualization of all aspects of the larynx. Then they introduce us to the nuances of contact microendoscopy. The photographic illustrations are magnificent and add clarity to the accompanying text and the clinical cases.

Dr. Andrea introduced contact microendoscopy to laryngologists throughout the world in 1994. This atlas further documents and demonstrates the promise of this innovative technique. It is sure to stimulate the design and development of new instrumentation and new assistive devices that will enhance visualization and control.

The possibility of using today's in vitro diagnostic studies to look at cellular biologic markers may well be extended to in vivo methodologies. This technique allows us the opportunity to bring molecular biologic tools to the operating room for real time analysis. One can imagine a technique being developed that would allow in vivo single cell analysis for the mutated p53 gene allowing a new field of cytosurgery to come into being.

Although this technique was first introduced by Hamou in 1983 to be used in gynecologic endoscopy, Andrea and Dias have shown great ingenuity in extending this technique's application. I believe there is great potential for contact microendoscopy in all areas of medicine. It is only a matter of time before we see new instrumentation, refinements of the technology of both lighting and optics (rigid and flexible), new capacities for controlled micromanipulation, as well as computer image analysis.

Andrea and Dias have made a seminal contribution to the field of laryngology and medicine at large. Now our individual and collective imaginations and ingenuity can build from their foundation. Patients for generations to come will benefit from the fine, pioneering work of these two physician scientists.

Michael E. Johns, M.D.
Dean of Medical Faculty
Vice President for Medicine
Johns Hopkins University School of Medicine
Baltimore, Maryland

Acknowledgments

The publication of this Atlas would not be possible without the kind support of friends and institutions who gave their invaluable assistance in the development of rigid and contact endoscopic techniques.

We thank Dr. Michael Johns for his stimulating support and for the honor of having written the Foreword to this Atlas. We also appreciate the friendly and caring support given by Dr. Haskins Kashima to this project. For the development of rigid and contact endoscopy, we recognize Dr. William Ritchmeister, Dr. Marshall Strome, Dr. Robert Ossoff, Dr. Marvin Fried, and Dr. James Kelly.

Our gratitude goes to the staff and residents of the Department of Otolaryngology of the Faculty of Medicine of the University of Lisbon/Hosptial de Santa Maria, especially Dr. Alberto Santos and Dr. Carlos Macor, and to the anesthesiologists who helped us develop REMS and CEMS techniques. Thanks are also extended to the nursing, audiovisual, and clerical staffs of the department, all of whom contributed to this Atlas. The work performed during the last years at the Otolaryngology Research Center of the University of Lisbon (JNICT) has been fundamental as a source of many of the ideas developed in this publication.

We also recognize the Gulbenkian Foundation for the continuous support given to the implementation of new medical technologies in our department throughout the years, and the Luso-American Foundation, which allowed the collaboration between the Department of Otolaryngology of the Faculty of Medicine of Lisbon and institutions and departments of otolaryngology and head and neck surgery in the USA.

We thank Karl Storz and its representative in Portugal (Centro Tecnico Hospitalar) for their support to the Department of Otolaryngology at the University of Lisbon in the development of rigid and contact endoscopy in microlaryngeal surgery. We also thank Canon for their interest; and Reproscan, whose help in image processing was fundamental to the first phase of this book.

Finally, we thank Lippincott - Raven Press, and particularly Ms. Kathey Alexander and Ms. Joyce-Rachel John, for their assistance and support with this Atlas.

Clinical Cases

1

Introduction

As the ability to endoscopically assess the larynx has progressed, so has the field of laryngology. Manuel Garcia, in 1854, was the first to describe visualization of the vocal cords with a mirror. In the 1960s, Kleinsasser proposed the technique of suspension microlaryngeal surgery as it is practiced today. In recent years, videoendoscopic assessment (rigid endoscopy, fiberoptic endoscopy, stroboscopy, and videomicrolaryngoscopy) has significantly influenced diagnosis, treatment, and follow-up of patients with laryngeal pathology.

Studies of laryngeal morphology (1–6) have emphasized the need to observe the larynx from different perspectives in order to improve the assessment of pathology. In particular, the anterior commissure, the ventricle, the subglottis, and the inferior surface and free border of the vocal cord must be made visible (Figs. 1,2). However, the endoscopic techniques generally available in the office and the operating room limit the observation of the vocal cord to its superior surface. This hampers not only the diagnosis and treatment of the disease, but also the physician's understanding of the underlying pathophysiology of the disease (23,27,35,40,45).

Studies with laryngostroboscopy (27) have underlined the importance of the free border of the vocal cord. At this moment, a clear definition of its extent does not exist. Anatomic descriptions, based on cadaver studies, define the vocal cords as transverse folds with superior and inferior surfaces. But, according to stroboscopy, the free border of the vocal cord should be considered a dynamic anatomic area, corresponding to the most superior part of the inferior surface, and the shapes in this area are constantly changing during phonation, coughing, and respiration.

A number of structural and pathophysiologic concerns motivated us to develop the techniques discussed in this Atlas, including:

1. the fact that the major blood supply of the vocal mucosa, including the superior surface, originates at the subglottis from branches of the middle anteroinferior laryngeal artery which penetrates the larynx through the cricothyroid ligament;

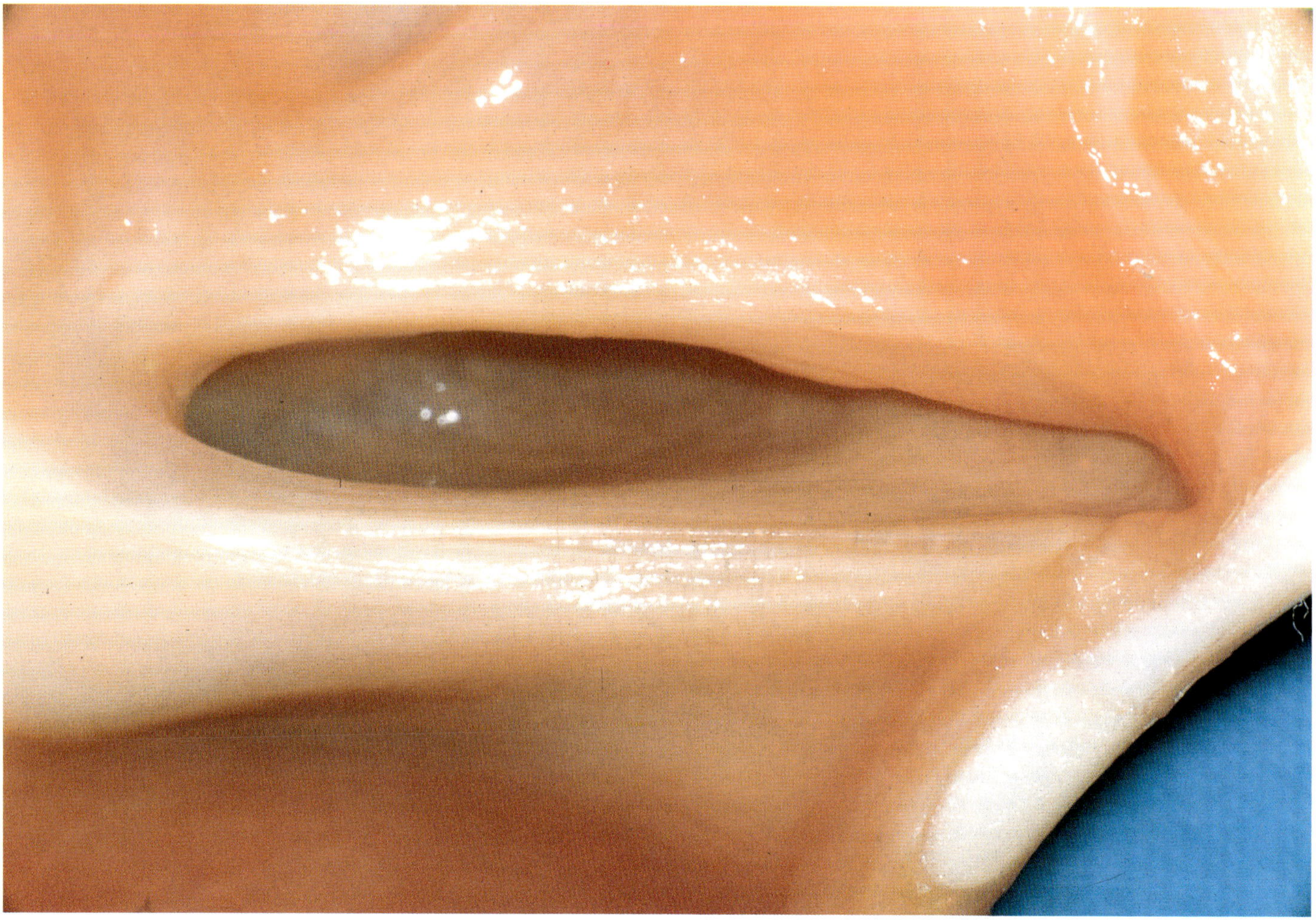

FIG. 1. Larynx photographed after sectioning of the thyroid cartilage. The vocal cord (superior surface, free border, and inferior surface), the anterior commissure, the arytenoid, the ventricle, the false cord, and the subglottis can be seen.

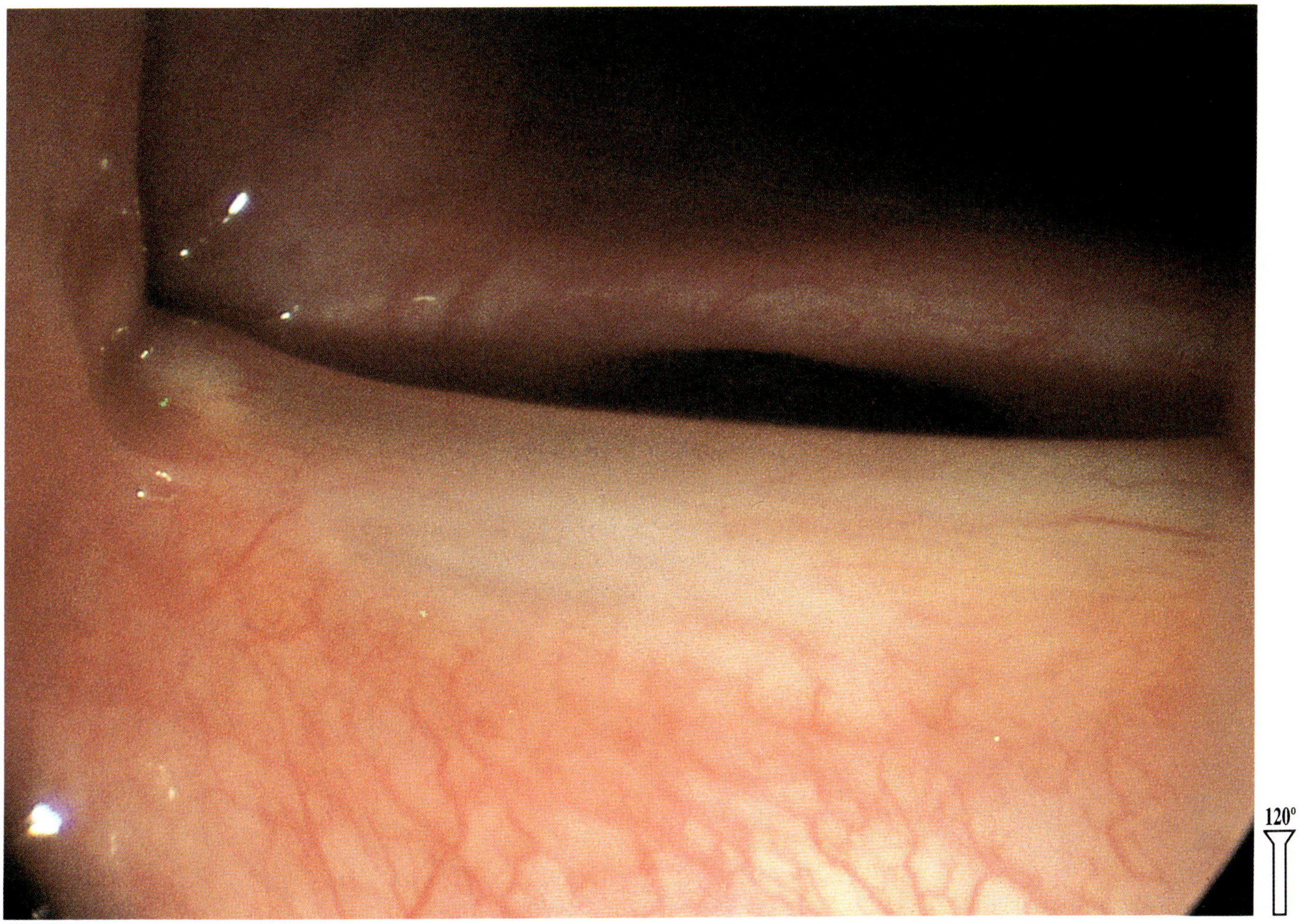

FIG. 2. Image of the inferior surface and free border of the vocal cord obtained with a rigid endoscope (120°) during microlaryngoscopy.

2. the importance of the elastic skeleton of the larynx at the level of the subglottis and the easy dissociation of the vocal ligament from the rest of the conus elasticus;
3. the fact that the inferior vocal cord surface is subjected to greater mechanical trauma than the superior surface;
4. the need to assess the inferior surface and subglottic extension of vocal cord tumors.

The use of endoscopy for subglottic assessment of laryngeal tumors by the technique of transconioscopy was proposed by Martensson et al. (33). The use of rigid endoscopy during microlaryngoscopy is practiced and advocated by Lehmann et al. (31), Benjamin (16–18), and Kleinsasser (29,30). However, in the majority of cases, its use has been restricted to the enhancement of access in the vertical axis (43).

Videomicrolaryngoscopy was proposed by Kantor et al. (28). Although offering significant improvement in image quality (43,44), this technique still does not permit the observation of the inferior surface of the vocal cord and subglottis.

Therefore, we began to use rigid endoscopes with different angles of vision (0°, 30°, 70°, and 120°) during microlaryngoscopies with the patient under general anesthesia. The quality of the images obtained and the access to areas that formerly could not have been assessed encouraged us to routinely perform Rigid Endoscopy during Microlaryngeal Surgery (REMS) (7–14). REMS is a natural evolution of the techniques of microlaryngoscopy and laryngeal endoscopy. It is safe and easy to perform, and the equipment it requires, with the exception of the telescopes, is currently available in most departments.

The observation of the vocal cords with the lens of a rigid endoscope positioned a few millimeters off the lesion rather than through the surgical microscope alone (with a focusing distance of 400 mm) allows a wider field of vision, increased depth of field, improved illumination, better image resolution, a higher magnification, and, in general, an improved definition of the images. A rigid endoscope also provides topographic localization, with access to all regions of the endolarynx, even those formerly difficult or impossible to explore clinically. The telescope also allows the surgeon to observe a particular lesion or region from different angles, allowing for multiperspective, three-dimensional reconstruction of the lesion (38).

REMS, which is based on a knowledge of laryngeal microanatomy, improves the assessment of all forms of laryngeal pathology. Parameters important in the evaluation of premalignant and malignant lesions can be analyzed in greater detail. REMS also benefits benign pathology: techniques of phonosurgery (instrumental or CO_2 laser) may be modified after assessment with REMS.

Contact Endoscopy performed during Microlaryngeal Surgery (CEMS) is the second technique presented in this Atlas. It has been developed in sequence with REMS, using a microcolpohysteroscope (Hamou I), and it brings a new dimension to the observation of the endolarynx, allowing the study of the epithelium in "real time" (Fig. 3).

With contact endoscopy, magnifications of 60° and 150° are used to study the superficial layers of the epithelium previously stained with methylene blue, *in vivo* and *in situ*. These magnifications allow direct access to the cells and to their characteristics. Several parameters can be evaluated: regularity of the epithelium, dimensions and color of the nucleus, nucleus/cytoplasm ratio, nuclear and cytoplasmic contours, and the presence of nucleoli, mitoses, cytoplasmic inclusions, keratosis, and koilocytes.

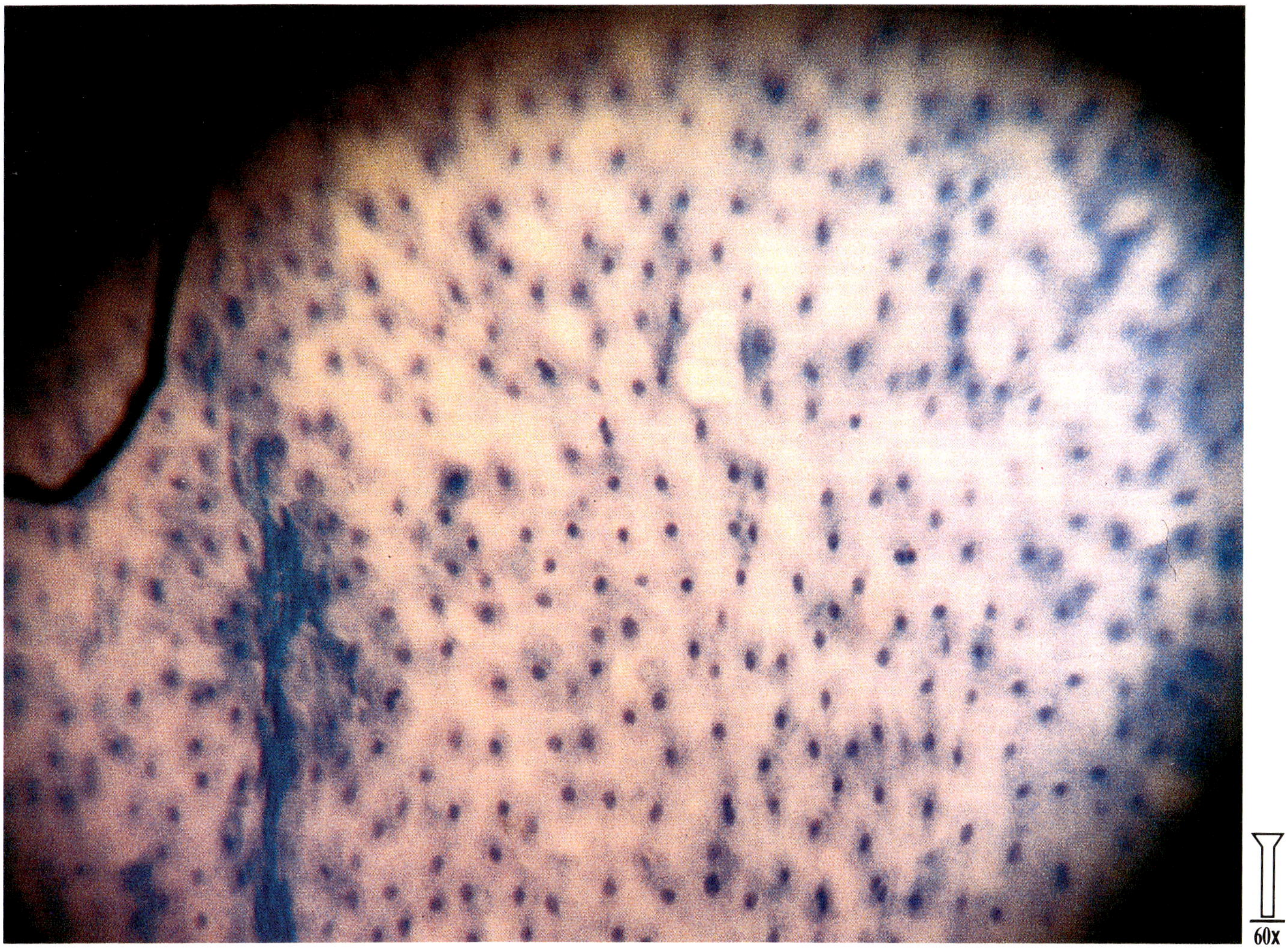

FIG. 3. Vocal cord epithelium observed by contact endoscopy. Squamous epithelium is visualized after methylene blue staining. A homogeneous cellular pattern [nucleus (dark blue) and cytoplasm (light blue)] can be seen on the superior surface of the vocal cord (60×).

Although biopsy is the best way to assess the depth of a lesion, the mobility of the contact endoscope permits the mapping of cellular alterations over the entire mucosal surface, documenting normal squamous epithelium (with a homogeneous cell arrangement, spheroid and isochromic nuclei, and a regular nucleus/cytoplasm ratio), to patterns specific for pathology such as chronic laryngitis, keratosis, dysplasia, papilloma, and malignant tumor. Furthermore, this technique also permits the observation of the microvascular network of the mucosa (7–14).

Further developments in contact endoscopy will increase its diagnostic capabilities and allow improved understanding of several physiopathological processes. The correlation of contact videoendoscopy images with morphologic techniques for surface assessment will also improve its diagnostic possibilities. Contact endoscopy may add significantly to the study of angiogenesis in inflammation, infection, malignancy, and healing (21,22,24,32).

The articulation of clinical observation and pathological examination will be enhanced requiring a closer collaboration of the specialties. Both the laryngologist and the pathologist will need to be familiar with contact endoscopy. The accuracy of contact endoscopy will be enhanced with improvements of the optical

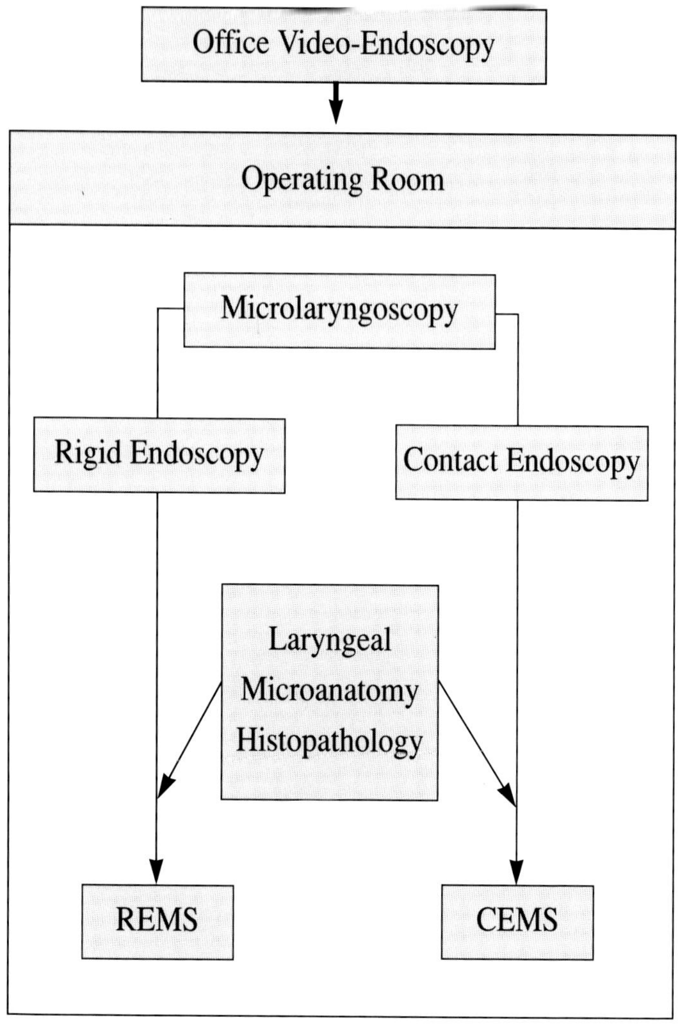

TABLE 1

systems, new cell dyes and markers (37), and better techniques of illumination, recording, and image processing. The first results with the prototype endoscope, which is being developed with Karl Storz, are very promising.

The potential of contact endoscopy in otolaryngology and head and neck pathology is enormous, with many clinical implications. Laryngology is an excellent field for the beginning of a new era of contact endoscopy, which in the future will be certainly applied to others specialties. Rigid and contact video endoscopy (Table 1) correspond to a new phase of development in laryngeal endoscopy and motivate a reflexion on physiopathology of the larynx on benign and malignant conditions. Further developments will be possible with the experience of different departments and institutions.

2

Techniques

RIGID ENDOSCOPY PERFORMED DURING MICROLARYNGEAL SURGERY (REMS)

Equipment (Table 2)

TABLE 2. *Rigid and Contact Endoscopy Equipment*

Endoscopes	5 mm; length 24 cm	
	Karl Storz 8712AA	0°
	Karl Storz 8712BA	30°
	Karl Storz 8712CA	70°
	Karl Storz 8712DA	120°
Contact endoscopes	Karl Storz Hamou I - 26156 B, 4mm	
	Karl Storz Prototype Contact Laryngoscope 8715A	
Light source	Karl Storz Xenon Light Source 615	
	Karl Storz—TTL Flash Unit	
Video	Camera—Karl Storz CCD 9050	
	S-VHS-Video recorder JVC RH G810V	
Photography	OM-40 zoom 70-140 mm	
	Ektachrome 100 ASA 35 mm	
Chest support	Karl Storz 8575 GK	
Autostatic support	Karl Storz 723018	

Suspension microlaryngoscopy is performed using conventional Kleinsasser laryngoscopes, selected on the basis of patient's age. An operating microscope is used with adaptors for video and photographic cameras.

Currently, rigid endoscopes (5 mm; length, 24 cm) with different angles of vision (0°, 30°, 70°, and 120°) are used (Karl Storz 8712 AA, 8712 BA, 8712 CA, and 8712 DA). In the early phase of the project, 4 mm endoscopes were used. Now, in the evaluation of some stenosis and tumors, endoscopes with 4 mm (or even lower caliber) may be indicated.

Videoendoscopic assessment is performed using a Xenon light source (Karl Storz 615), a video camera (Karl Storz CCD 9050), and an S-VHS video recorder (JVC RH-G810V). Slides (Ektachrome 100 ASA, 35 mm) are obtained using a camera (Olympus OM 40) connected to an electronic flash unit (Karl Storz, TTL).

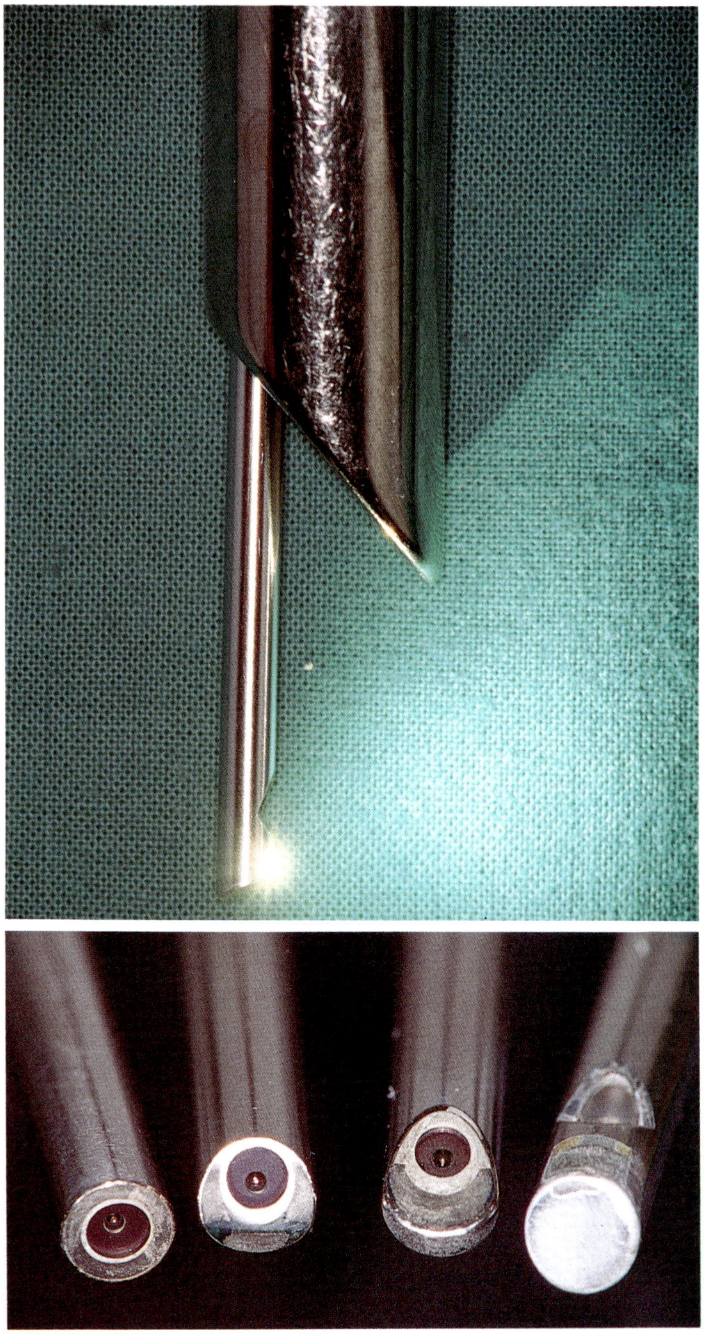

FIG. 4. The telescopes are used through the laryngoscope. The use of rigid endoscopes with different angles (0°, 30°, 70°, 120°) allows access to all regions of the larynx. The telescopes offer superior image resolution, great depth of focus, and a wide field of vision.

Procedure

Anesthesia

In all patients, general anesthesia is performed with endotracheal intubation. The type and size of the tube are determined by the patient's age, the tracheal luminal size, and the planned surgical technique (instrumental or CO_2 laser). Adults are preoxygenated with 100% oxygen, and intravenous droperidol and alfentanil are administered. Induction is initiated with intravenous propofol and maintained by endotracheal intubation and an infusion of propofol, atracurium, and alfentanil, with controlled ventilation. For microlaryngeal surgery, cuffed tubes with a diameter between 4 and 6 mm are used. For CO_2 laser microlaryngeal surgery, appropriate tubes of the same caliber are used.

In children, inhalation anesthesia is performed utilizing cuffless tubes.

REMS

The laryngoscope is positioned, taking into account the site of the lesion, and the tip of the laryngoscope is visualized with a 70° endoscope. The laryngoscope is suspended using a Riecker-Kleinsasser holder and chest support (Karl Storz 8575 GK). First, the larynx is observed with the microscope at several magnifications. Then the endolarynx is inspected using the endoscope at 0°, 30°, 70°, and 120°.

Following a careful assessment, the microsurgical excision or biopsy of the laryngeal lesion is performed and the site is reassessed with the telescopes.

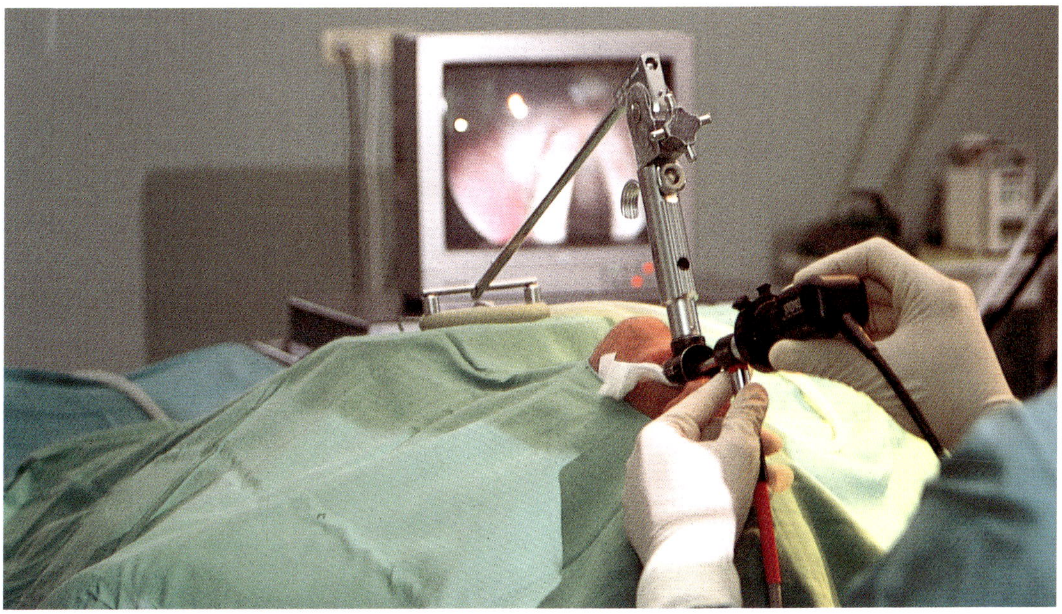

FIG. 5. REMS is performed under conventional general anesthesia with endotracheal intubation. Videoendoscopic assessment of benign, premalignant, and malignant pathology is performed with 0°, 30°, 70°, and 120° telescopes during microlaryngoscopy.

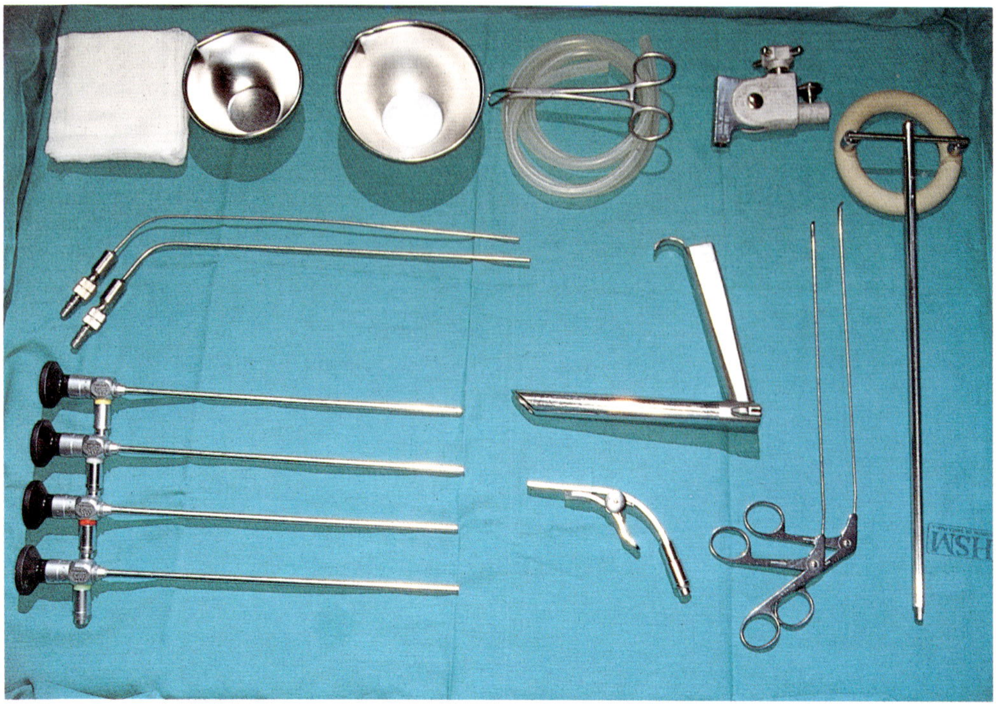

FIG. 6. Instrument table for REMS and CEMS, equipped with laryngoscope, light clip, chest holder, telescopes (0°, 30°, 70°, 120°), contact endoscope, aspiration tube and cannulas, microlaryngeal forceps, and containers of methylene blue, saline serum, anti-fog solution, gauze, and Spongostan.

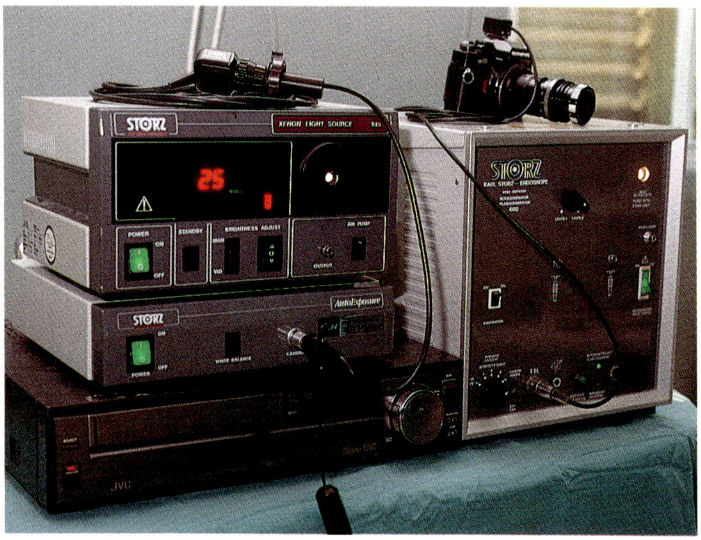

FIG. 7. Imaging equipment includes K.S. Xenon light source, K.S. TTL flash unit, photographic camera (OM 40) with zoom lens (70–140 mm), video camera K.S. CCD 9050, video recorder S-VHS JVC RH G810V.

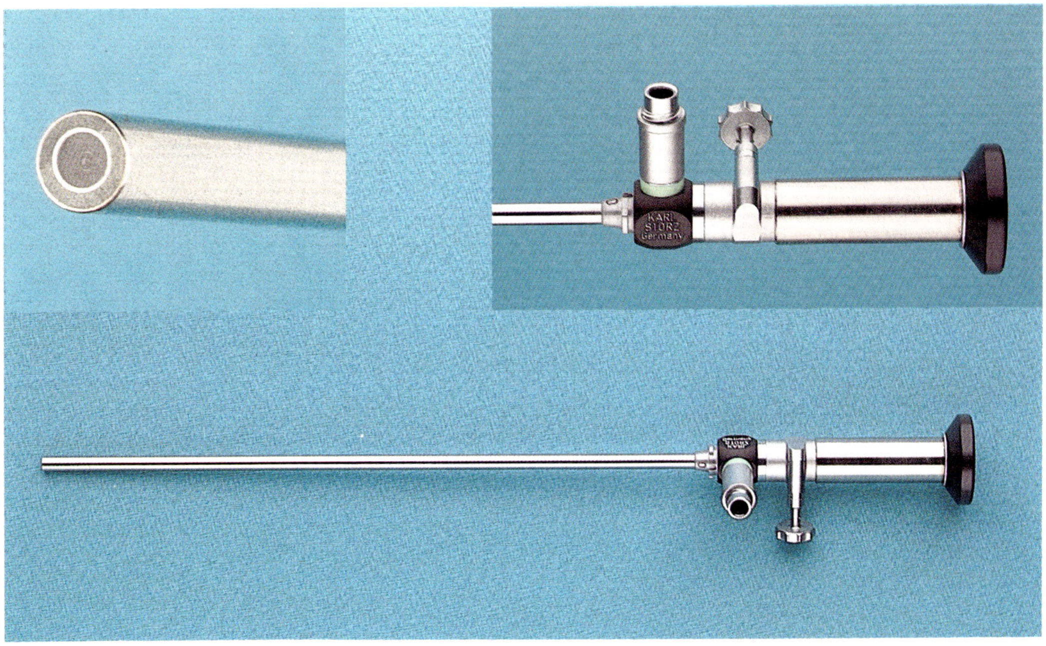

FIG. 8. Contact laryngoscope K.S. 8715A.

CONTACT ENDOSCOPY DURING MICROLARYNGEAL SURGERY (CEMS)

Equipment (Table 2)

For contact videoendoscopy, we start with a microcolpohysteroscope (Hamou I-Karl Storz 26156B), 24 cm long, 4 mm in diameter, with an angle of 30°. When in contact with the tissues, it allows for magnifications of 60° and 150° (25,26,39). Presently, a prototype developed in collaboration with Karl Storz is being used (contact laryngoscope—K. S. 8715A).

Contact endoscopy is performed after the assessment with the microscope and the telescopes. An autostatic device (Karl Storz 723018) fixed to the operating table improves the manipulation of the contact endoscope, allowing for better control of movement along the superior surface of the vocal cord. Video and photographic documentation are obtained with the same equipment used in REMS.

Procedure

With the contact endoscope close to the mucosal surface, allowing a panoramic view, the superior surface of the vocal cord is cleaned using Spongostan soaked in saline serum. After careful suction of the area, the vocal cords are stained with 1% methylene blue.

The mucosa is gently touched with the tip of the contact endoscope, and the stained cells of the superficial layers of the epithelium become visible. The color lasts for approximately 4 to 5 minutes and gradually disappears, so staining is repeated periodically if longer assessment of the epithelium is needed.

Later, contact videoendoscopic images are compared with histologic sections of the biopsied or excised lesions. Video recording allows for study and discussion of the images obtained by this *in vivo* and *in situ* study of the tissues.

3

Patients

Three hundred and forty three patients who underwent microlaryngoscopy over 2 years were studied with rigid endoscopy performed during microlaryngeal surgery (REMS). Of these, 240 were male patients and 103 were female. Their ages ranged from 2 years to 83 years, with a mean of 51 years. In 145 patients, contact endoscopy (CEMS) was also performed. Preoperatively, all patients were studied with videoendoscopy (90° and 70° rigid pharyngolaryngoscopes) and some with stroboscopy.

The pathologies studied were malignant tumors, polyps, leukoplakia, chronic laryngitis, Reinke's edema, juvenile papillomatosis, papillomas, subglottic stenosis, nodules, vocal cord cysts, contact granulomas, ventricular eversion, vocal cord synechiae, larynx after irradiation, histoplasmosis, trauma, postintubation granuloma, bilateral vocal cord paralysis, sulcus glottidis, and tuberculosis (Table 3).

TABLE 3. *Patients studied by REMS and CEMS*

DIAGNOSIS	REMS	CEMS
Polyps	80	15
Nodules	7	-
Contact granulomas	3	-
Vocal cord cysts	8	5
Ventricle's eversion	3	-
Reinke's edema	16	10
Chronic laryngitis	37	22
Tuberculosis	1	-
Histoplasmosis	2	1
Juvenile papillomatosis	9	7
Papilloma	11	9
Trauma	2	-
Entubation granuloma	2	-
Vocal cord paralysis	2	-
Vocal cord synechiae	3	-
Subglottic stenosis	11	-
Sulcus glottidis	1	-
Leukoplakias	59	31
Malignant tumors	81	42
Larynx after radiotherapy	5	3
TOTAL	343	145

4

Results

Part I: REMS—Rigid Endoscopy Performed in Microlaryngeal Surgery

Topographic Assessment

The use of four endoscopes (0°,30°,70°,120°) improves the assessment of the endolarynx and neighboring regions, offering a multiperspective view of the lesions. The length (24 cm) and diameter (5mm) of the endoscopes allow observation of and access to the vocal cords during a routine endotracheal entubation.

Although the 0° telescope has an identical axis of vision as the microscope, it allows a far better resolution of the image and a wider field of vision, offering a detailed global vision of the superior surface of the vocal cords. Passing the cordal level, it gives access to the subglottis and trachea but misses important regions such as the free border and the inferior surface of the vocal cords.

The 30° telescope improves the visualization of the orifice and floor of the ventricle, allowing the observation of the anterior commissure from above. By rotating the endoscope the posterior commissure can also be evaluated.

But it is with the 70° and 120° telescopes that the endoscopic assessment of laryngeal pathology is greatly enhanced as critical areas in the clinical evaluation are exposed.

In the anterior midline, these endoscopes explore the laryngeal surface of the epiglottis, the epiglottic stem and the small region that separates it from the vocal

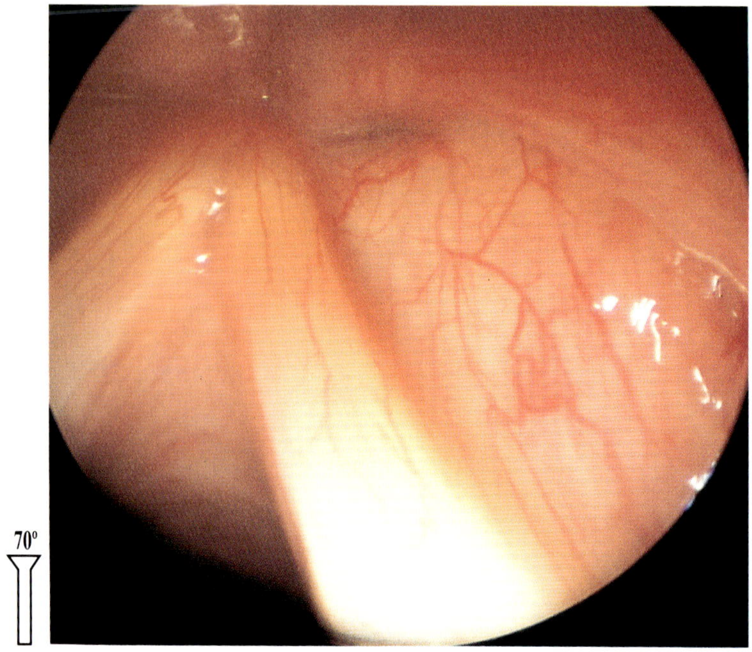

FIG. 9. Image of the superior surface of the vocal cord and ventricle obtained with a 70° rigid endoscope during microlaryngoscopy.

cords, the anterior commissure, the small slit between the vocal cords at the thyroid cartilage, the slim area of the free border of the vocal cords at the most anterior part, the subcommissural region, the area corresponding internally to the cricothyroid region, and the anterior part of the trachea.

Laterally, the 70° endoscope improves the visualization of the orifice and floor of the Morgagni ventricle, increasing our capacity to access its depth. Below the ventricle, the 70° endoscope positioned at the angle between the anesthesia tube and the vocal process of the arytenoid offers a superb view of the glottic margins in the horizontal and vertical planes. The height of the "free border", the relationship of the pathology on the opposite vocal cord, the inferior surface of the vocal cords, the mucosal characteristics and shape of the inferior part of the paraglottic space, as well as the tracheal mucosa are important benefits seen through a 70° telescope.

The 120° telescope permits backwards visualization of the superior limit of the ventricular orifice (false cord) and visualization of part of the vertical component of Morgagni ventricle. Rotation of the 120° telescope below the vocal cord offers a good view of the glott subglottic dome, including the subcommissural region, the inferior surface of the vocal cords and the small area below the base of the arytenoid cartilage.

Placing the 70° and 120° telescopes at the anterior part of the larynx and displacing the endotracheal tube, the posterior larynx can be observed; namely, the height of the arytenoid cartilages, the cricoarytenoid junction, the internal surface of the vocal process, the subarytenoid region, and the posterior part of the subglottis.

Each endoscope allows a specific perspective. The use of one or several endoscopes is determined by the anatomy and the characteristics of the pathology.

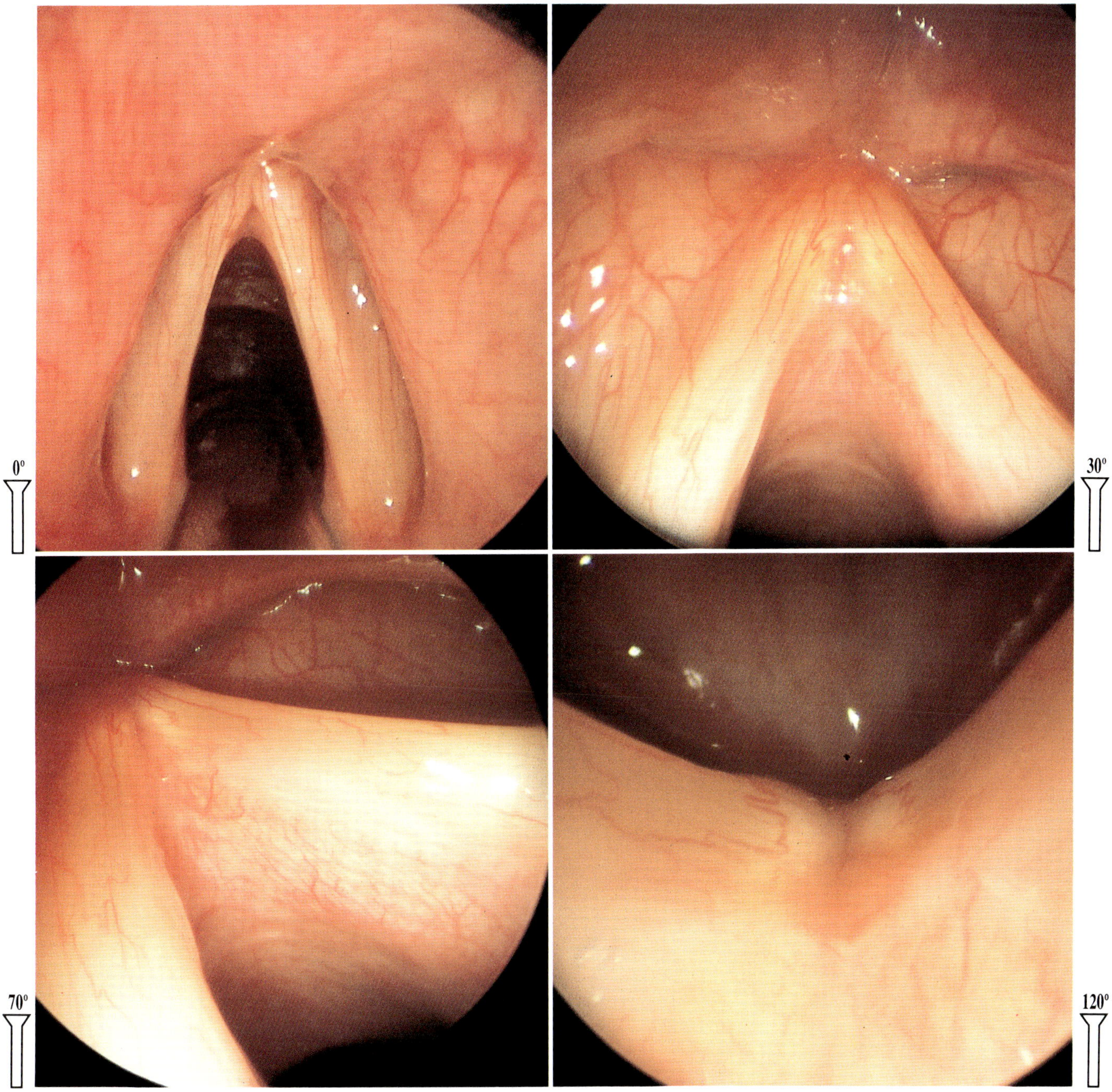

FIG. 10. REMS endoscopic assessment of the larynx. At the supraglottis, rigid endoscopy improves visualization of the laryngeal surface of the epiglottis, of the small zone that separates it from the vocal cords, and the opening of the ventricle.

At the glottis, the vertical dimension of the vocal cord at the free border and at the arytenoid region can be seen. The evaluation of the superior surface of the vocal cord during microlaryngoscopy is enhanced, as is the insertion of the vocal cord at the thyroid cartilage, its continuity to the ventricle, and the blood vessels and Reinke's space.

The length and height of the classic free border and the rest of the inferior surface of the vocal cord can be evaluated, whereas microscopic assessment of these regions is limited because of the axis of vision.

Note the definition of the subglottic mucosa, the lumen of the trachea, and the mucosa covering the first tracheal rings.

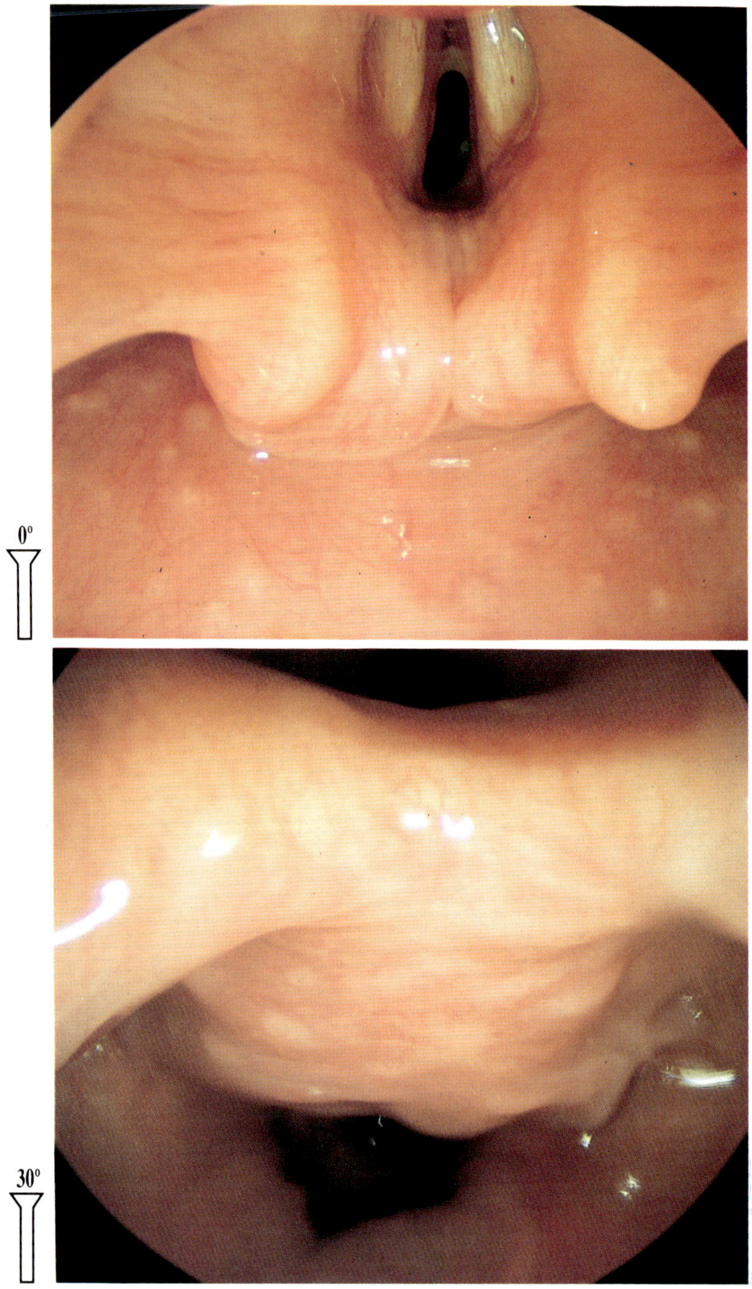

FIG. 10A. After the intubation tube is pushed to the front, the telescopes have access to the posterior region of the larynx and to the retrocricoid area.

Image Characteristics

The images obtained with the rigid endoscopes are of superior quality with greater depth of field and a wider field of vision than those obtained by surgical microscopy.

Image resolution is also better with the rigid endoscopy; this is particularly apparent at higher magnifications. At the same time, because rigid endoscopes can focus from a position very close to the lesion, the magnification is higher than that obtained with the microscope.

Multiperspective Assessment

Assessing a single lesion or a specific region of the larynx from different perspectives, or angles, allows for tridimensional evaluation of the pathology, whether benign, premalignant, or malignant. There is significant improvement of the definition and identification of the characteristics of the lesions (form, dimensions, boundaries, extension, color, relief, and vascular alterations) in all regions that can be observed with the surgical microscope, and in regions where inspection is difficult or even impossible in microlaryngoscopy.

BENIGN PATHOLOGY (Figs. 11–56)

When a polyp is observed with the surgical microscope, only its superior surface and the superior surface of the vocal cord can be assessed. Rigid endoscopy allows a more complete view of the polyp—its dimensions, localization, surface characteristics, and color, as well as the vasculature of the polyp and nearby zones. The inferior surface of the polyp and the dimensions of its base of implantation are clearly defined.

The multiperspective view of the base of implantation—horizontal and vertical axis—allows the surgeon to plan and to perform a meticulous surgical technique.

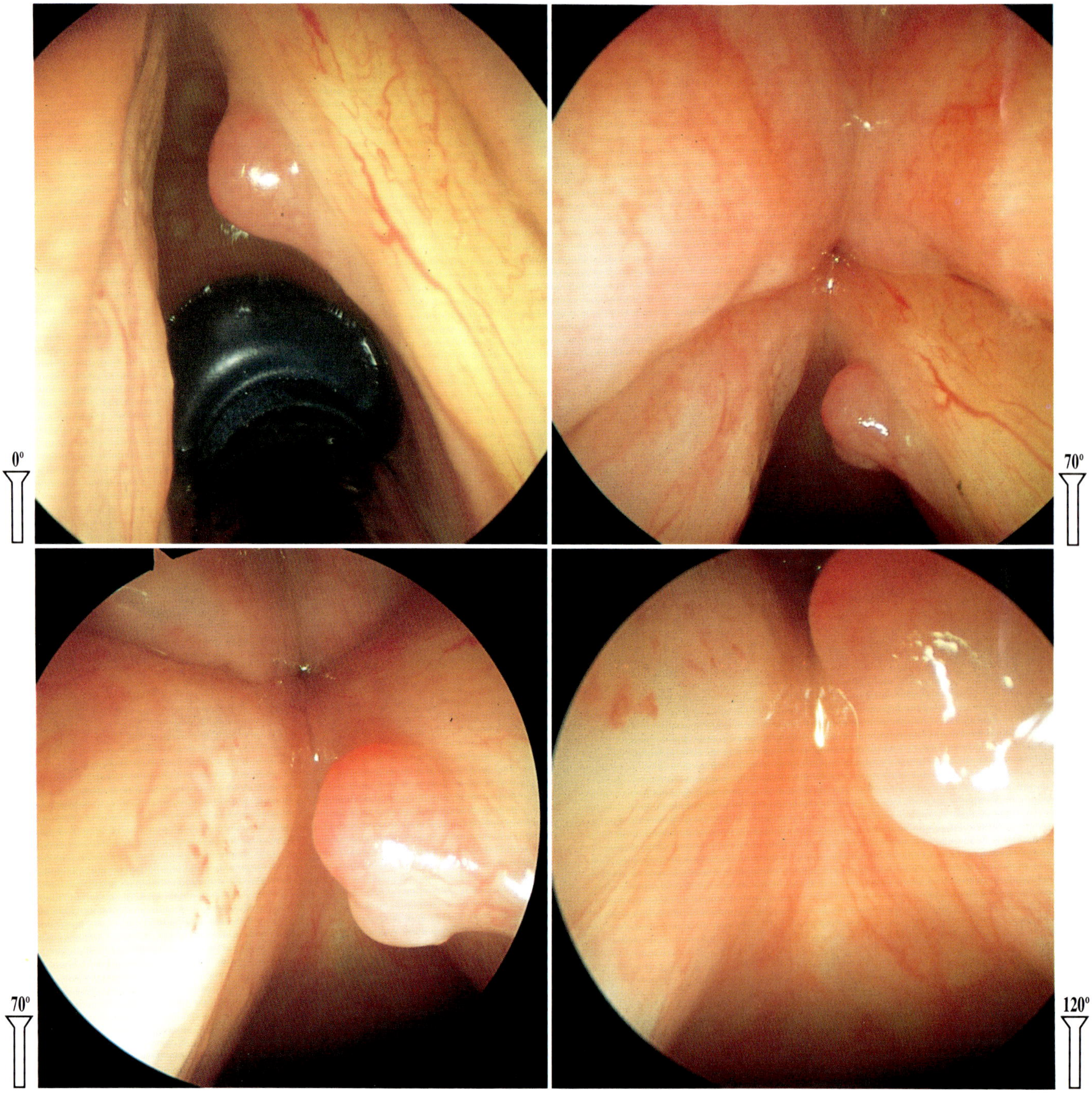

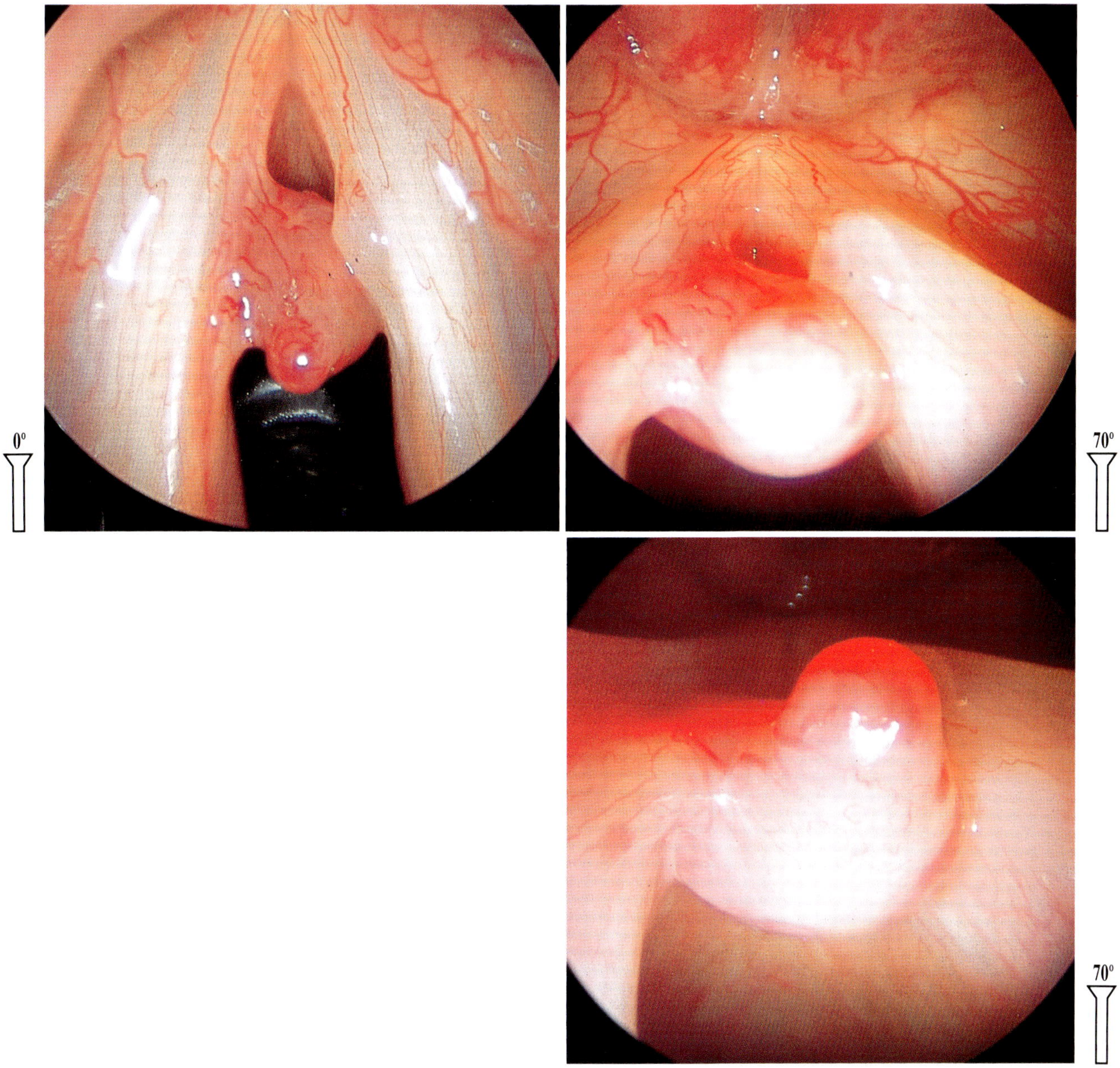

FIG. 12. This patient is a 35-year-old salesman with smoking habits. At the left vocal cord, there is a large hemorrhagic polyp. This polyp originates from the free border and inferior surface of the true cord. Its vasculature can be seen in detail. The base of implantation is evaluated with the different telescopes along its horizontal and vertical axes. On the right vocal cord, in addition to a smaller polyp, the mechanical trauma caused by the opposite lesion is observed.

FIG. 11. This patient is a 41-year-old man, a cigarette smoker and textile industry worker. There is a right vocal cord polyp with a large base of implantation at the inferior surface of the vocal cord. The superior surface of the polyp has a hemorrhagic appearance and its inferior surface is keratinized. In the contralateral cord, traumatic alterations can be identified: edema, a depression, telangiectasias, and keratinization. There are signs of inflammation in the glottic and supraglottic mucosa.

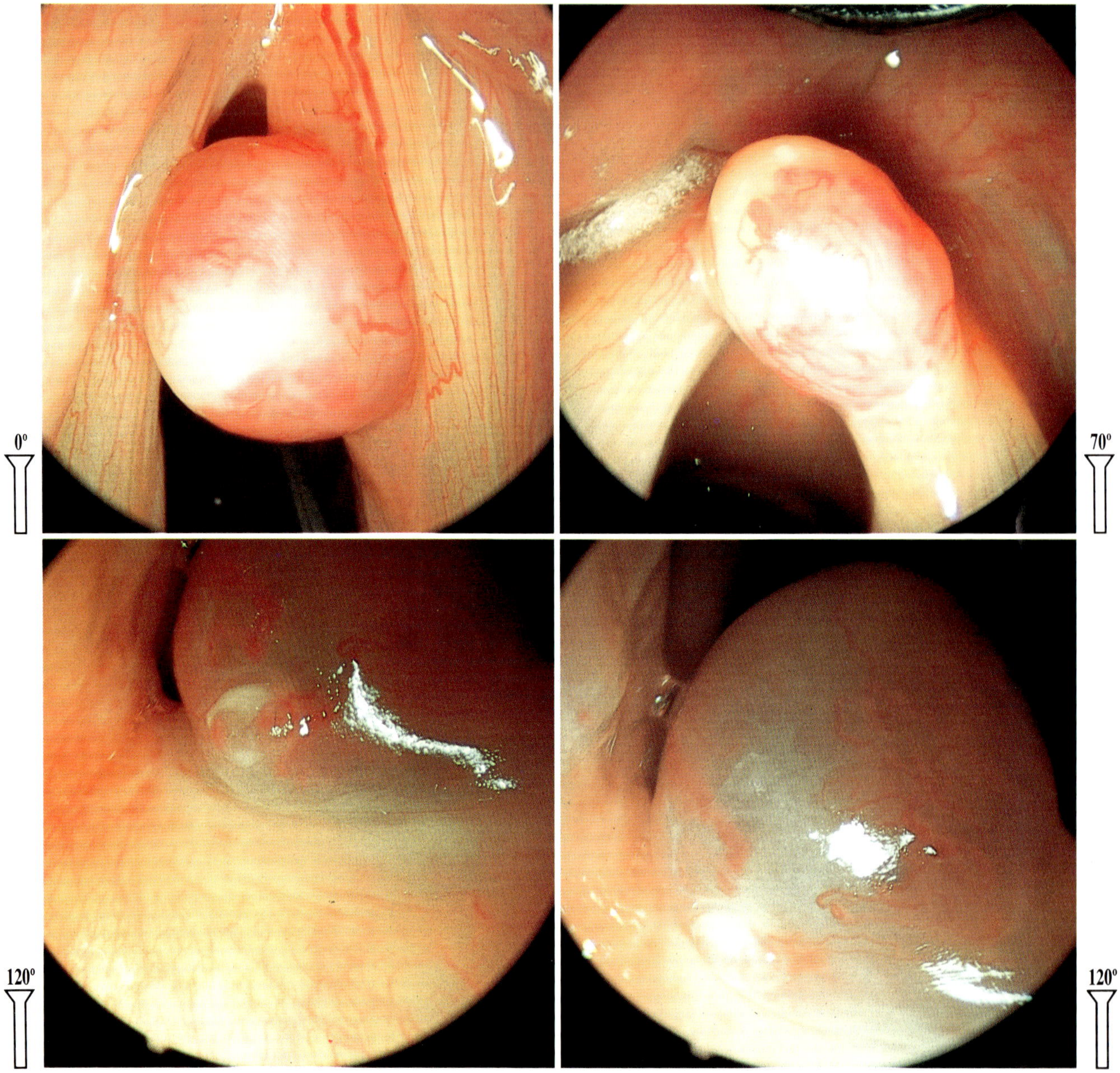

FIG. 13. This large polyp of the right vocal cord occurs in a 47-year-old industrial worker. The polyp has a hemorrhagic appearance with abnormal vasculature and areas of keratosis. The base is well-defined in its vertical axis and areas of edema are observed adjacent to the polyp. The 120° telescope allows the identification of a small area of keratosis at the inferior limit of the polyp. The increased vasculature of the vocal cord is clearly observed. The contralateral cord exhibits edema and keratosis.

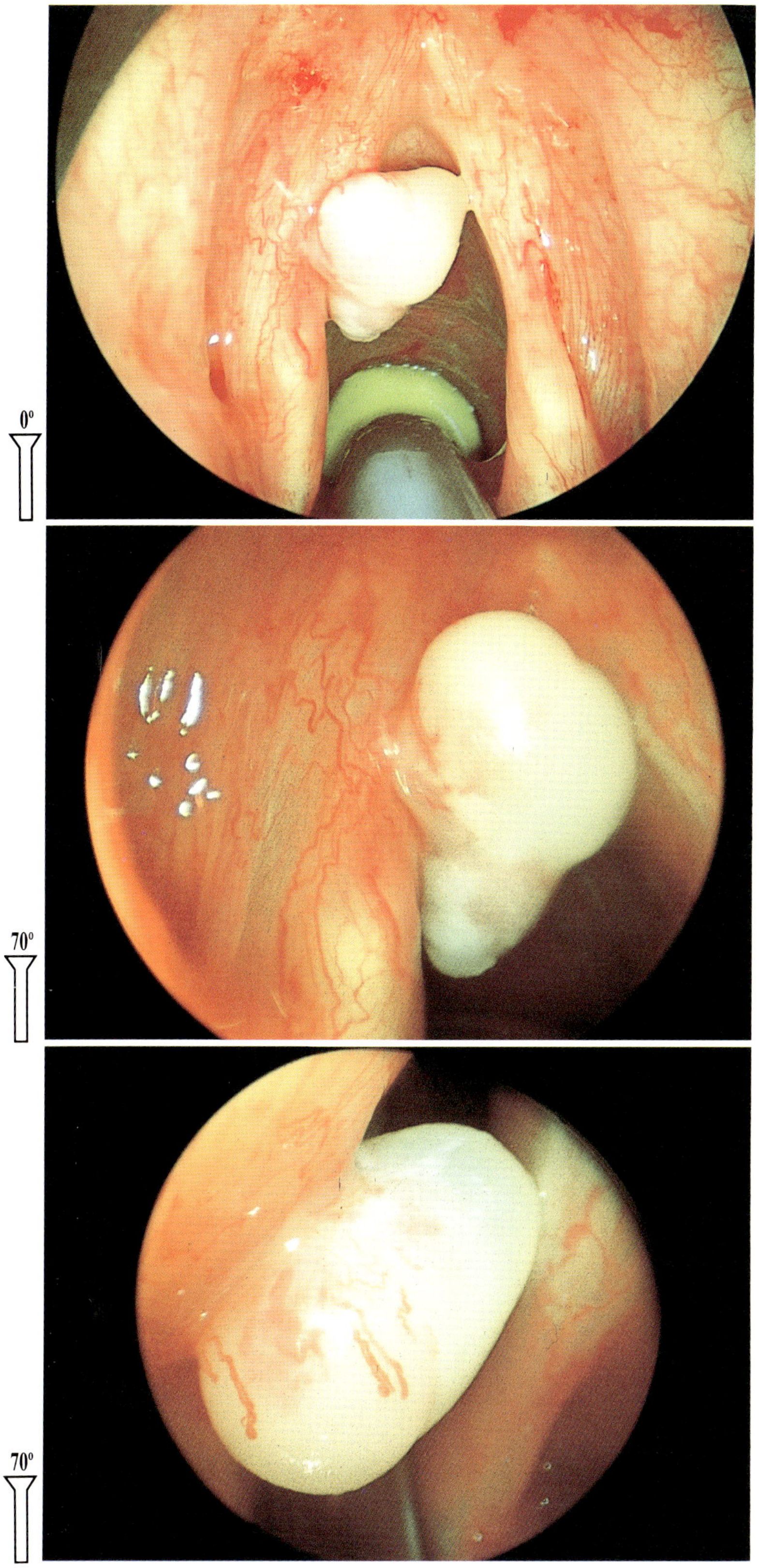

FIG. 14. This large whitish polypoid lesion was observed on the left true vocal cord in a 64-year-old shipyard worker. There is diffuse hypervascularity, particularly at the base. Observation of the lesion with the 70° telescope at the anterior commissure demonstrates vascular arcades suggestive of a papilloma. This diagnosis was subsequently confirmed on histologic examination.

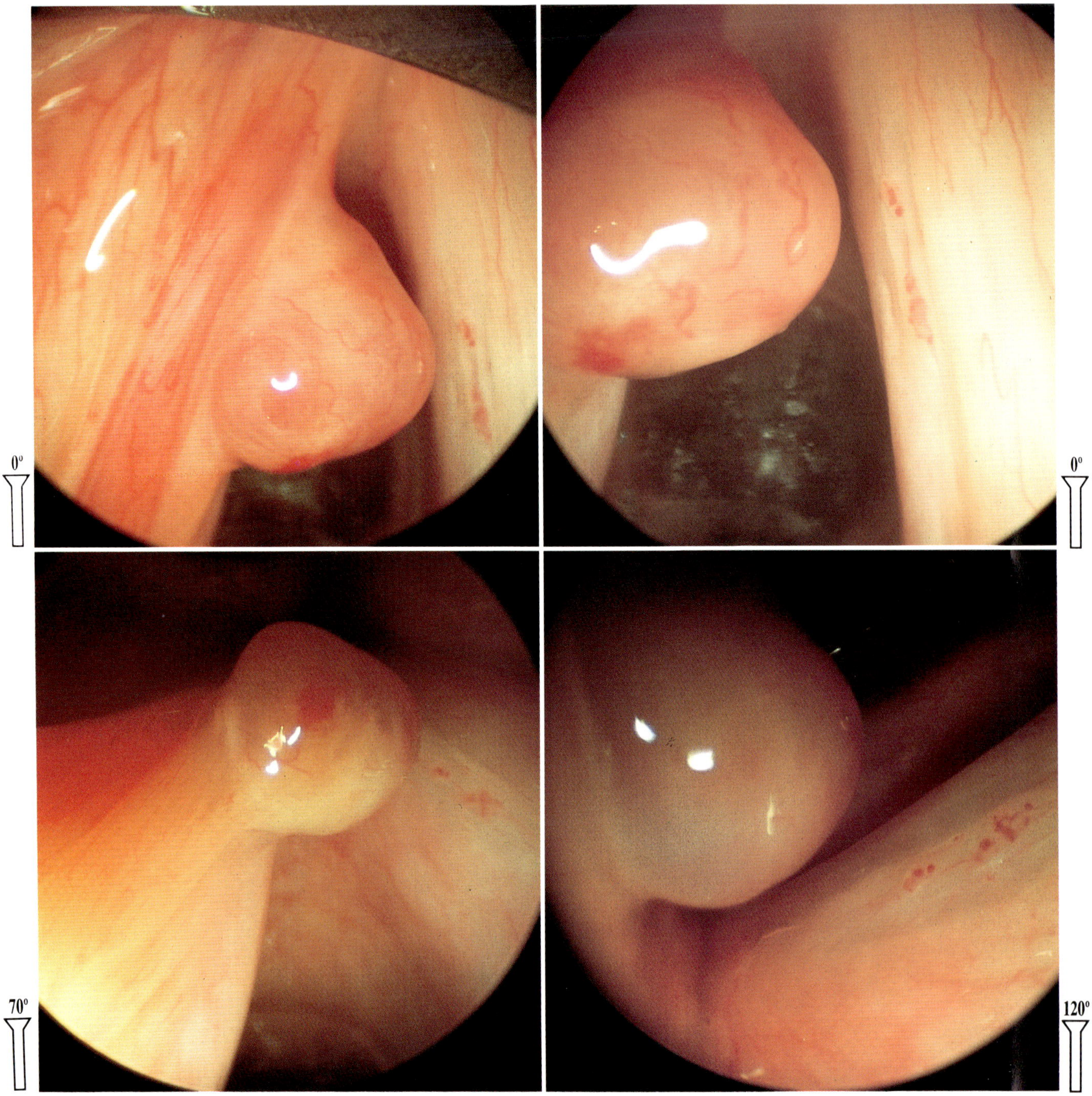

FIG. 15. This 36-year-old man is a cigarette smoker and an industrial worker. There is a large left vocal cord polyp with a hemorrhagic appearance. The superior surface of the vocal cord has increased vascularity and a hemorrhagic effusion. At the inferior surface of the polyp, the mucosa is keratinized. There is a large base of implantation at the free border. On the opposite vocal cord, traumatic contact alterations can be seen, such as keratinization and telangiectasias.

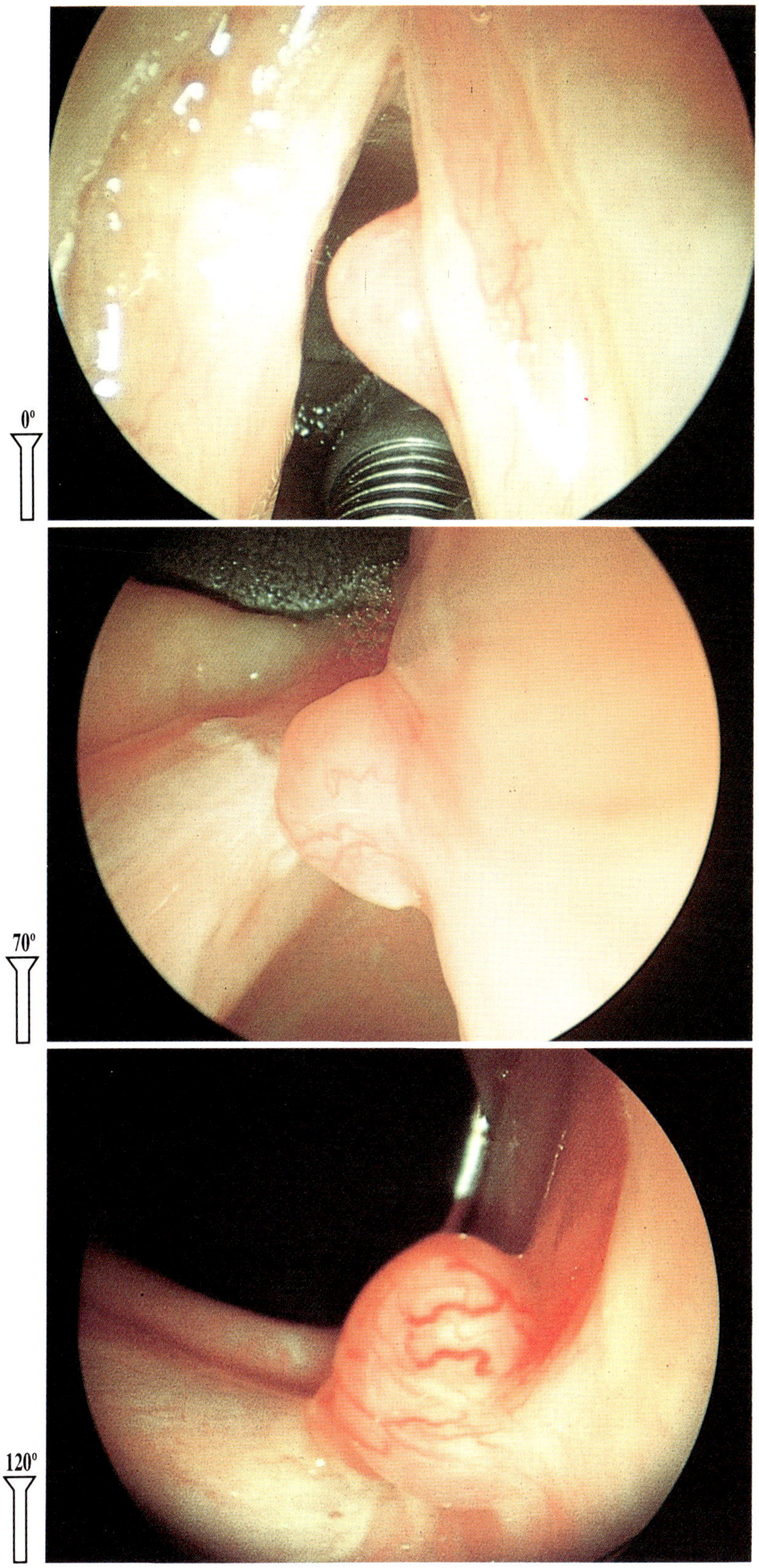

FIG. 16. This 51-year-old school teacher presents with a polyp at the right true vocal cord. The vertical axis of the base was evaluated with the 70° telescope and is comparable to the length in the horizontal axis. The 120° telescope allows observation of the inferior aspect of the polyp and its continuity with the inferior surface of the vocal cord. Note the edema and keratosis present bilaterally, but more pronounced on the contralateral cord, directly opposite the polyp.

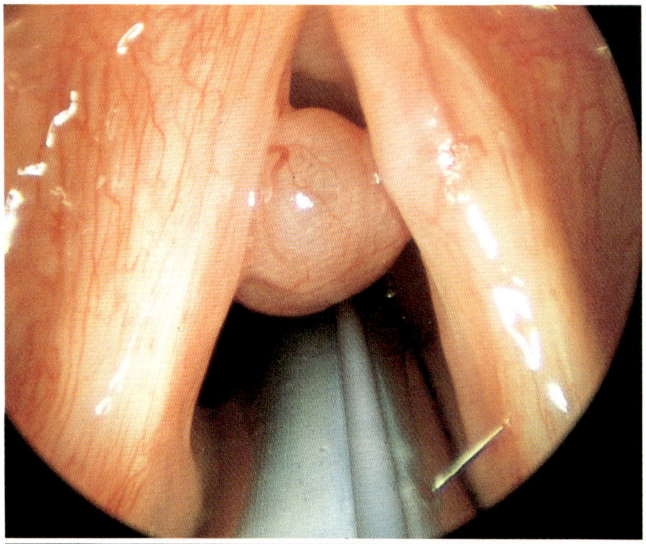

0°

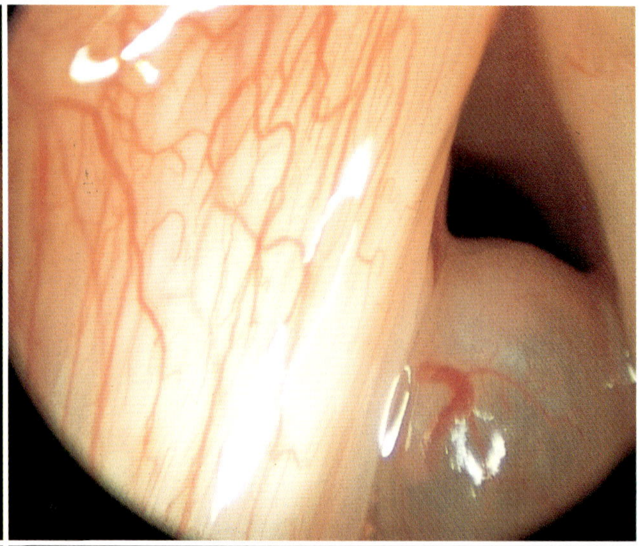

0°

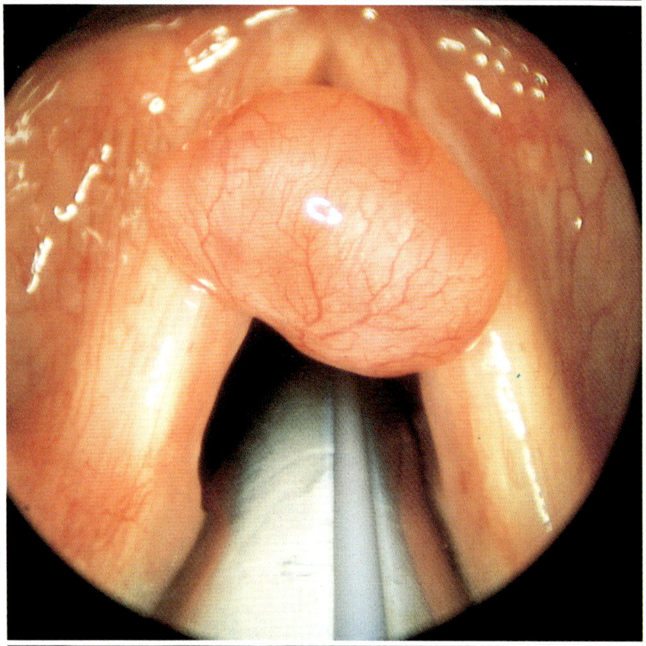

30°

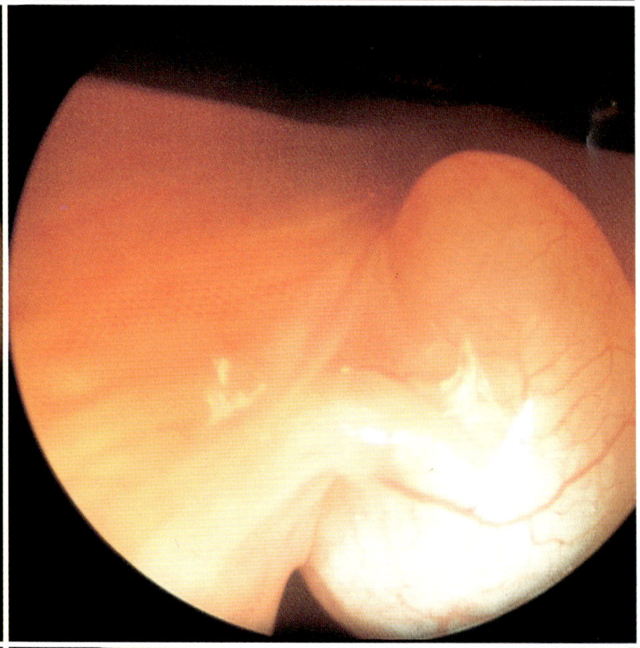

70°

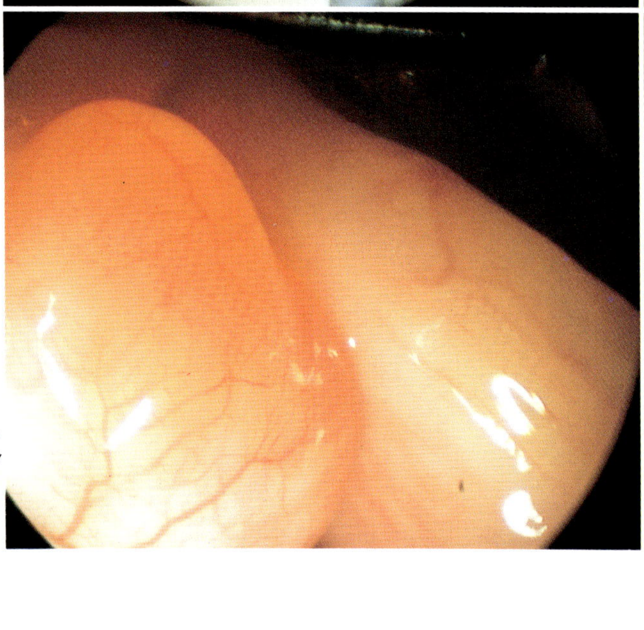

70°

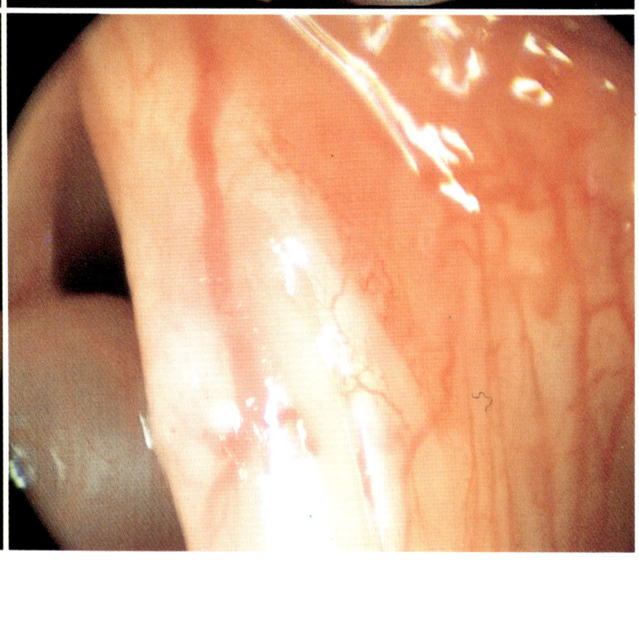

0°

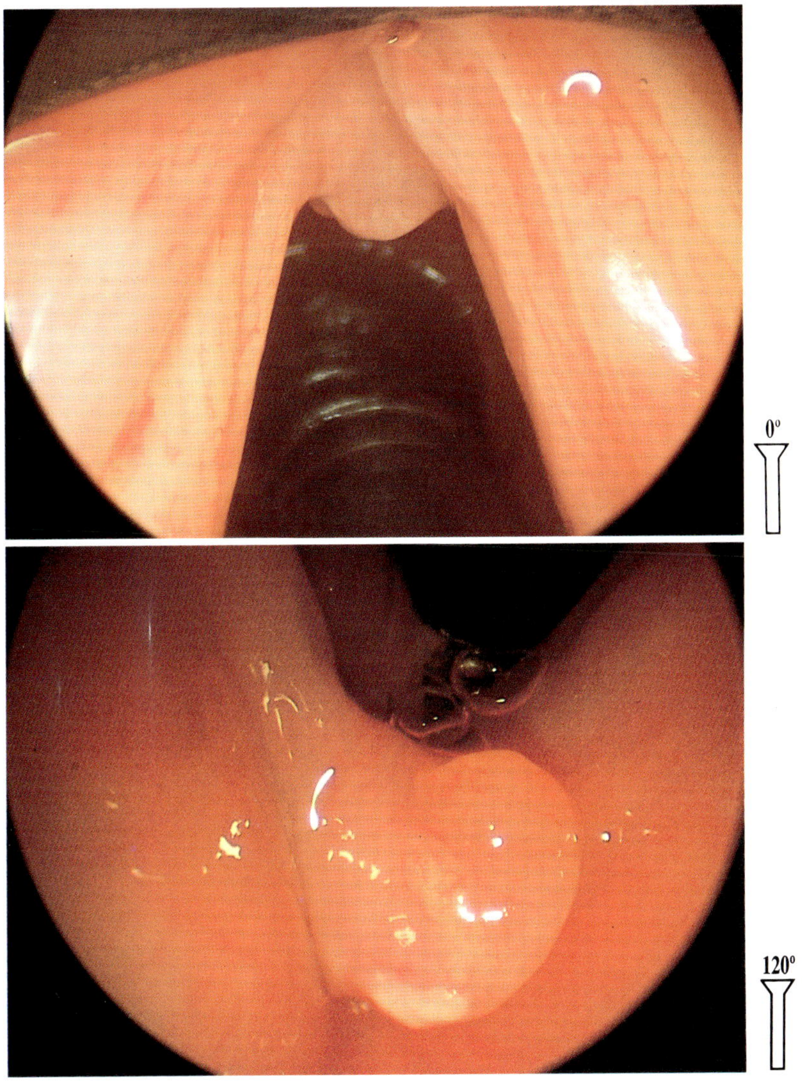

FIG. 18. This 57-year-old bus driver, with a history of smoking, exhibits a polyp at the anterior aspect of the left vocal cord. Using a 70° telescope, it is possible to clearly establish the characteristics of the polyp, including the origin of its base. Both vocal cords also demonstrate signs of chronic inflammation.

FIG. 17. This 39-year-old saleswoman has a large, pendulous, left vocal cord polyp with a base of implantation at the middle one-third of the vocal cord, originating from its inferior surface. On the opposite cord, there is a keratinized surface. The degree of keratinization still allows observation of blood vessels through the leukoplakia.

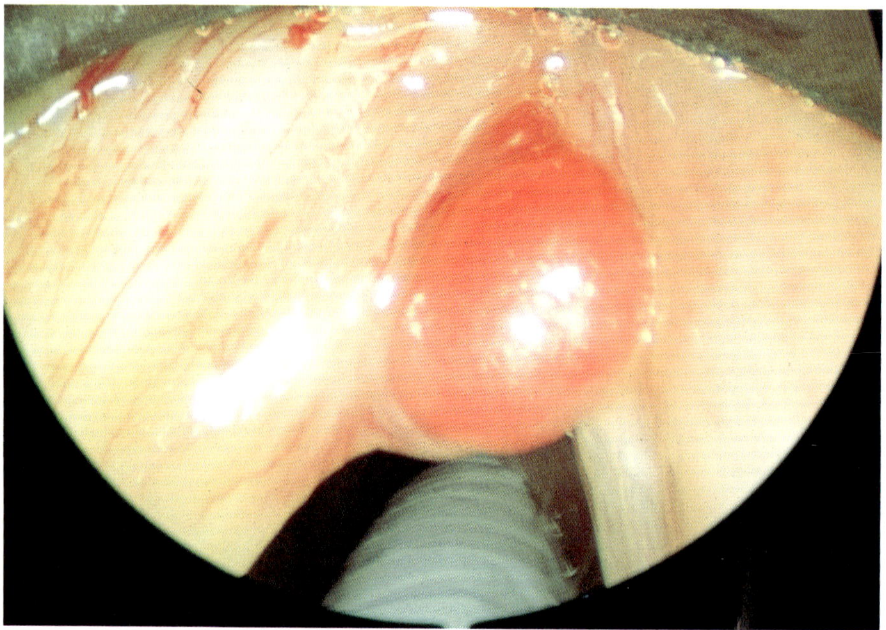

0°

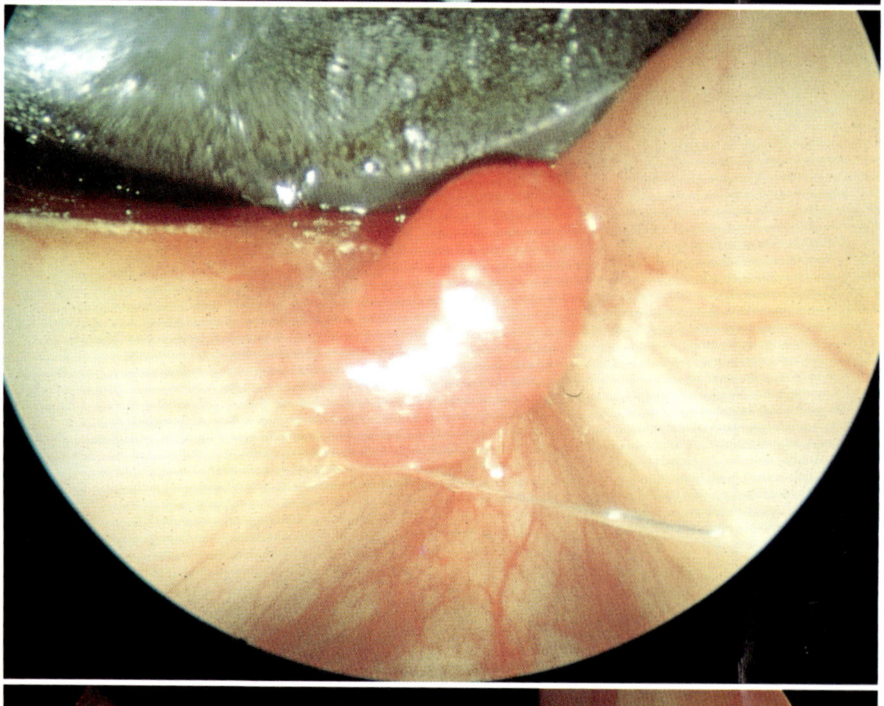

70°

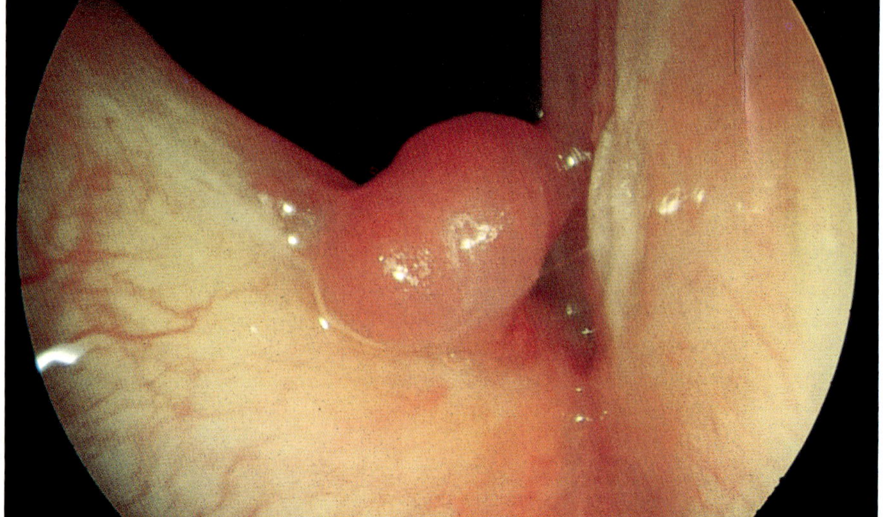

120°

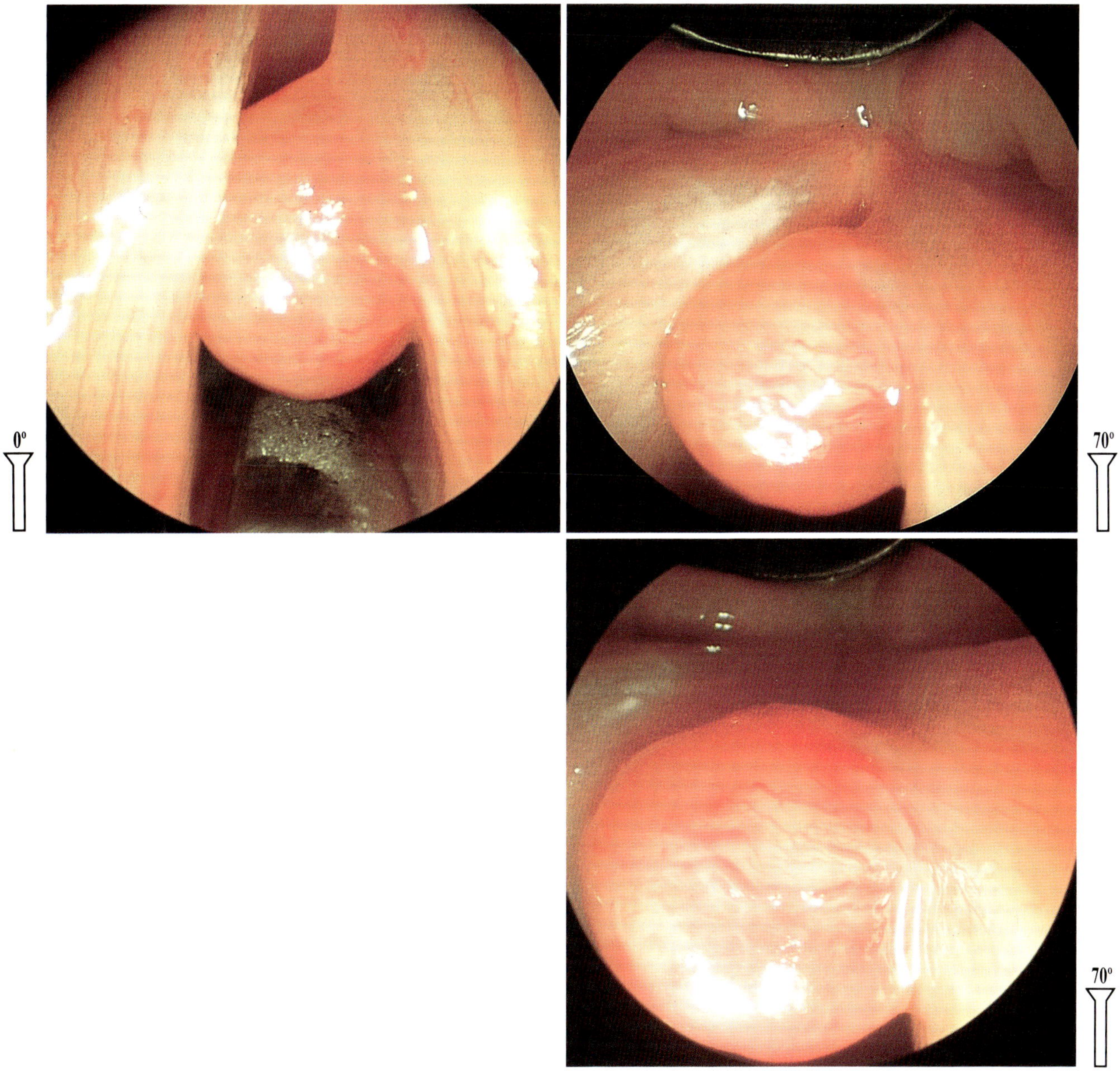

FIG. 20. This 45-year-old textile worker presents with a large, broad-based polyp of the right vocal cord, originating from the free border and inferior cordal surface. Disturbed vasculature as well as traumatic alterations (edema and keratosis) are visualized on both sides of the larynx.

FIG. 19. This 55-year-old man is a cigarette smoker and cereal warehouse worker. He has a hemorrhagic polyp of the anterior part of the left vocal cord with a thick base of implantation at the free border and inferior surface of the vocal cord. Keratinization is particularly evident at the inferior surface and at the contact area of the opposite vocal cord. Diffuse edema of both vocal cords is noticed at the superior surface.

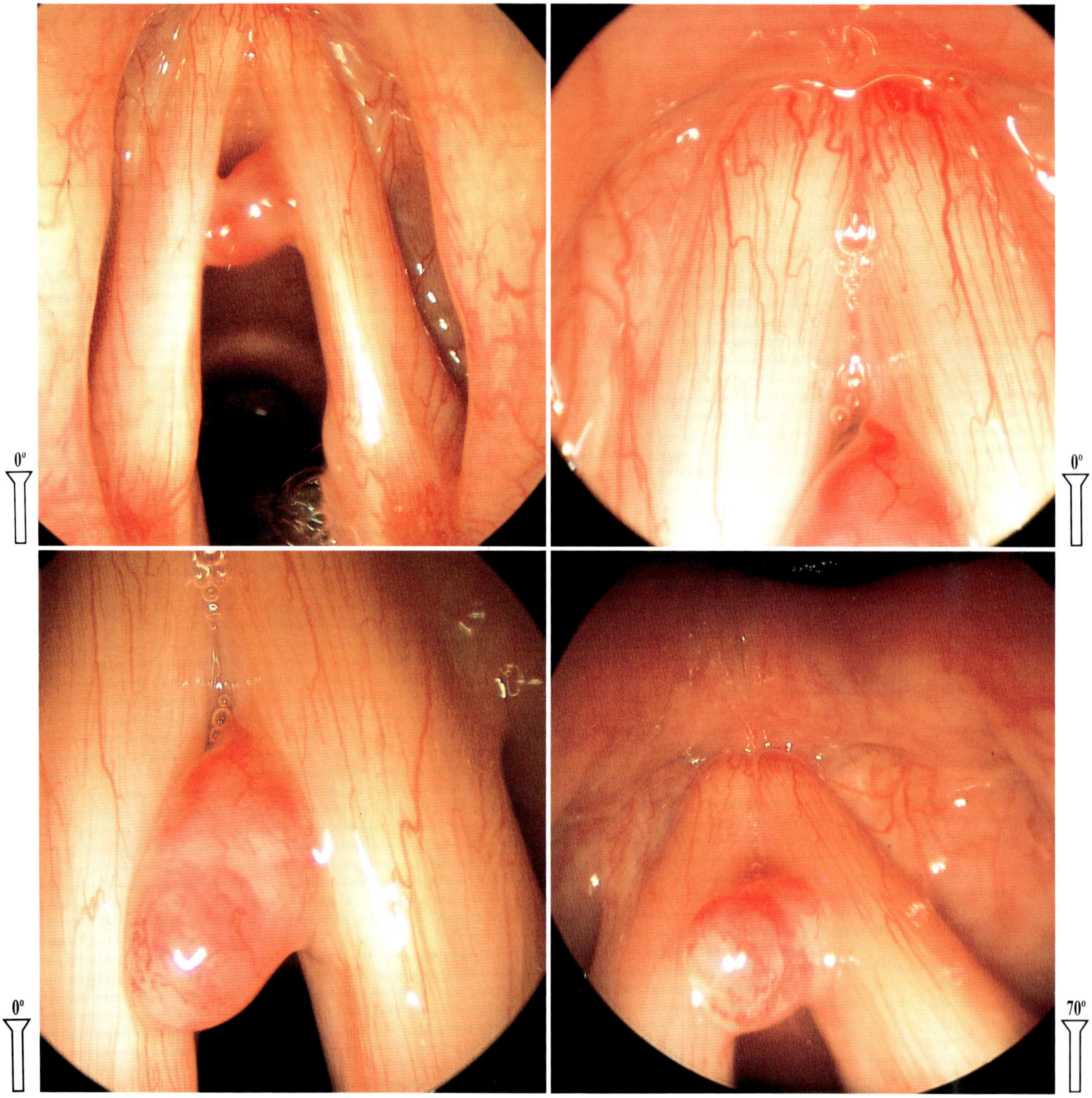

FIG. 21. This 32-year-old man is a high school teacher with a hemorrhagic polyp of the right vocal cord. The vasculature of the superior surface of the vocal cord is not disturbed. The base of implantation is situated at the free border.

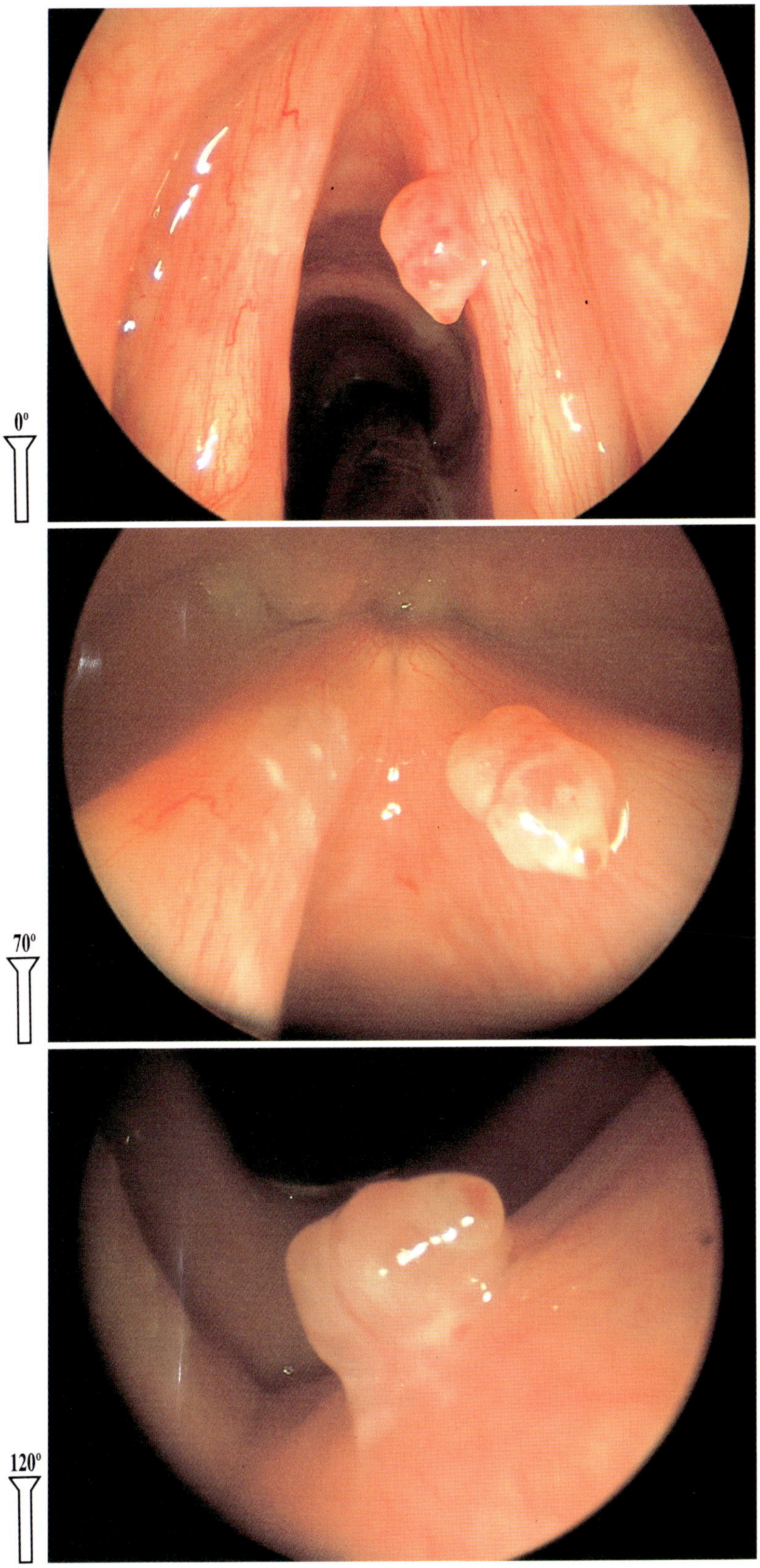

FIG. 22. Examination of this 59-year-old bank employee with smoking habits reveals a polyp at the right true vocal cord. Keratosis is again seen on a small area along the opposite vocal cord. The endoscope allows a detailed evaluation of the site, size, and surface characteristics of the polyp.

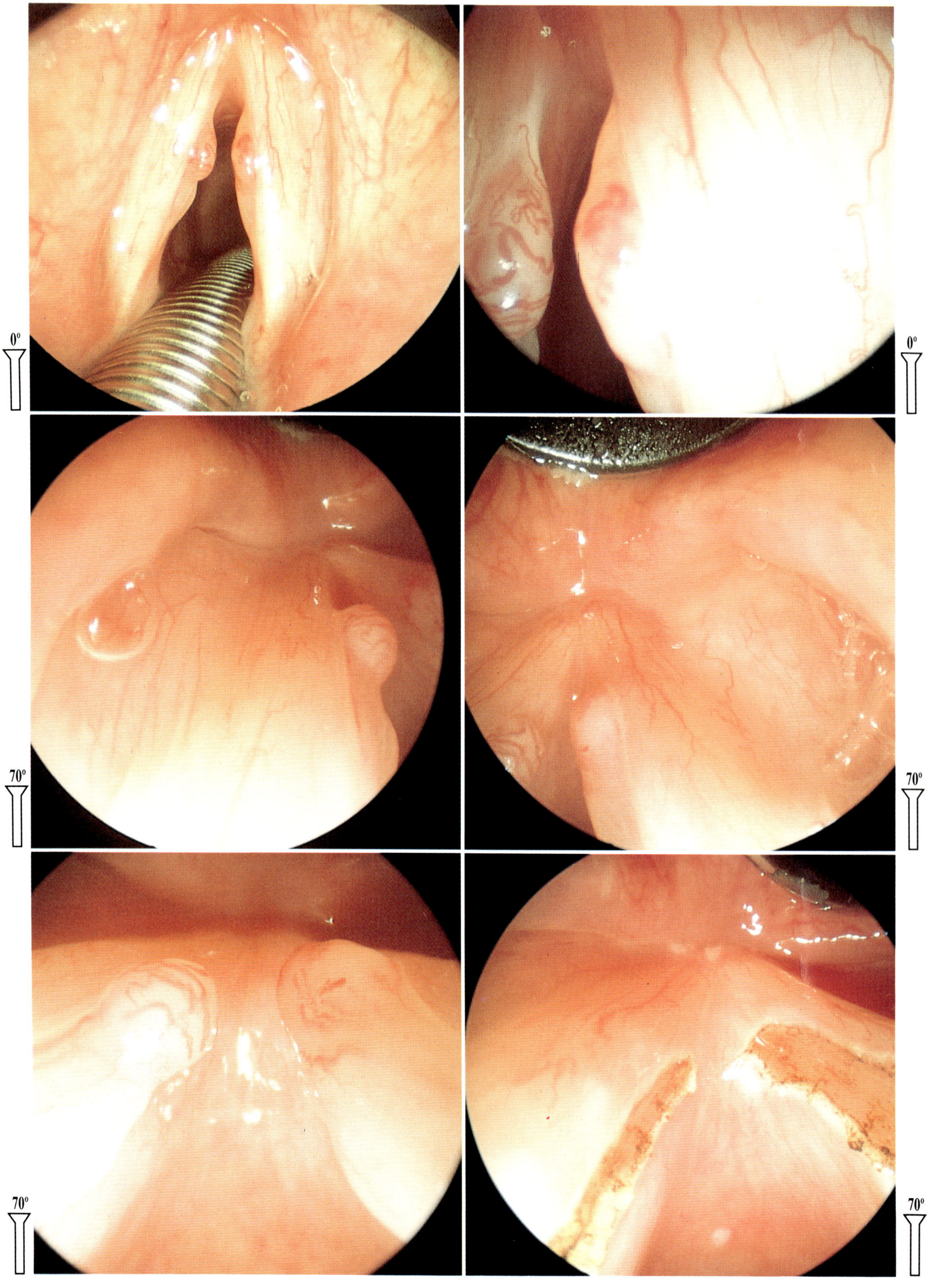
0°
0°
70°
70°
70°
70°

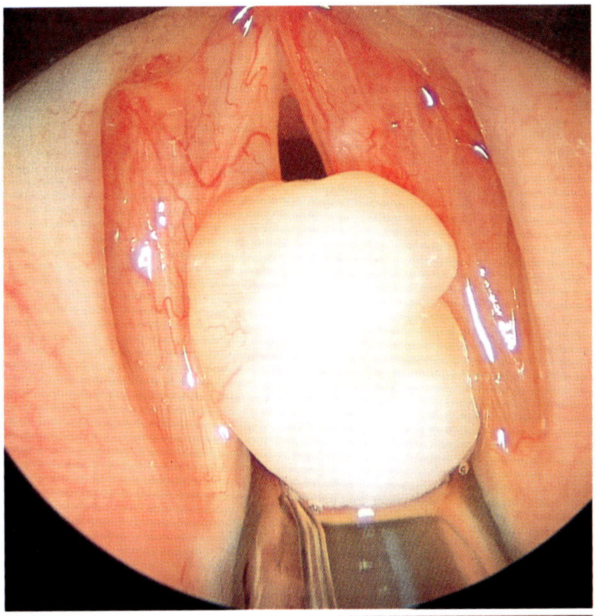

0°

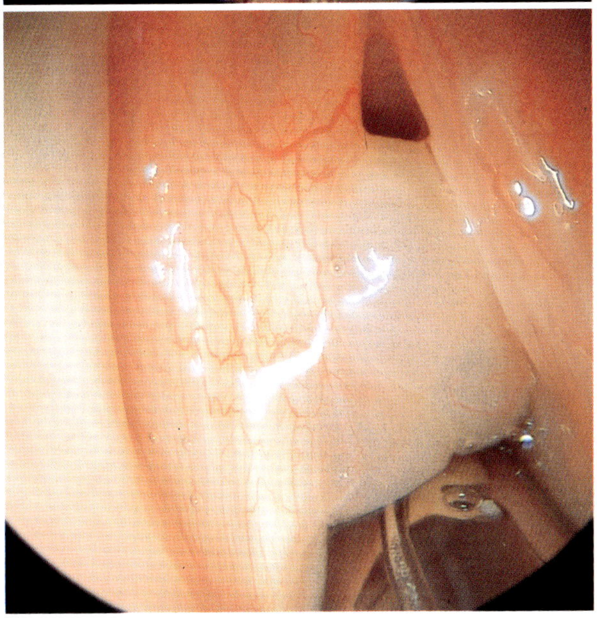

0°

FIG. 24. This large polyp of the left vocal cord occurs in a 27-year-old teacher. The vasculature of both vocal cords is disturbed secondary to the lesion and its contralateral traumatic effect. On the right vocal cord, an area of keratosis is seen.

FIG. 23. This 40-year-old woman is an industrial worker. She has bilateral, symmetric polyps with gelatinous appearance. Vascular abnormalities are apparent. The base of implantation is situated at the free border of the vocal cords. Anterior and posterior areas of edema extend along the base of implantation along the free border of the vocal cords. After CO_2 laser microsurgery, the area of exeresis is observed with the 70° endoscope.

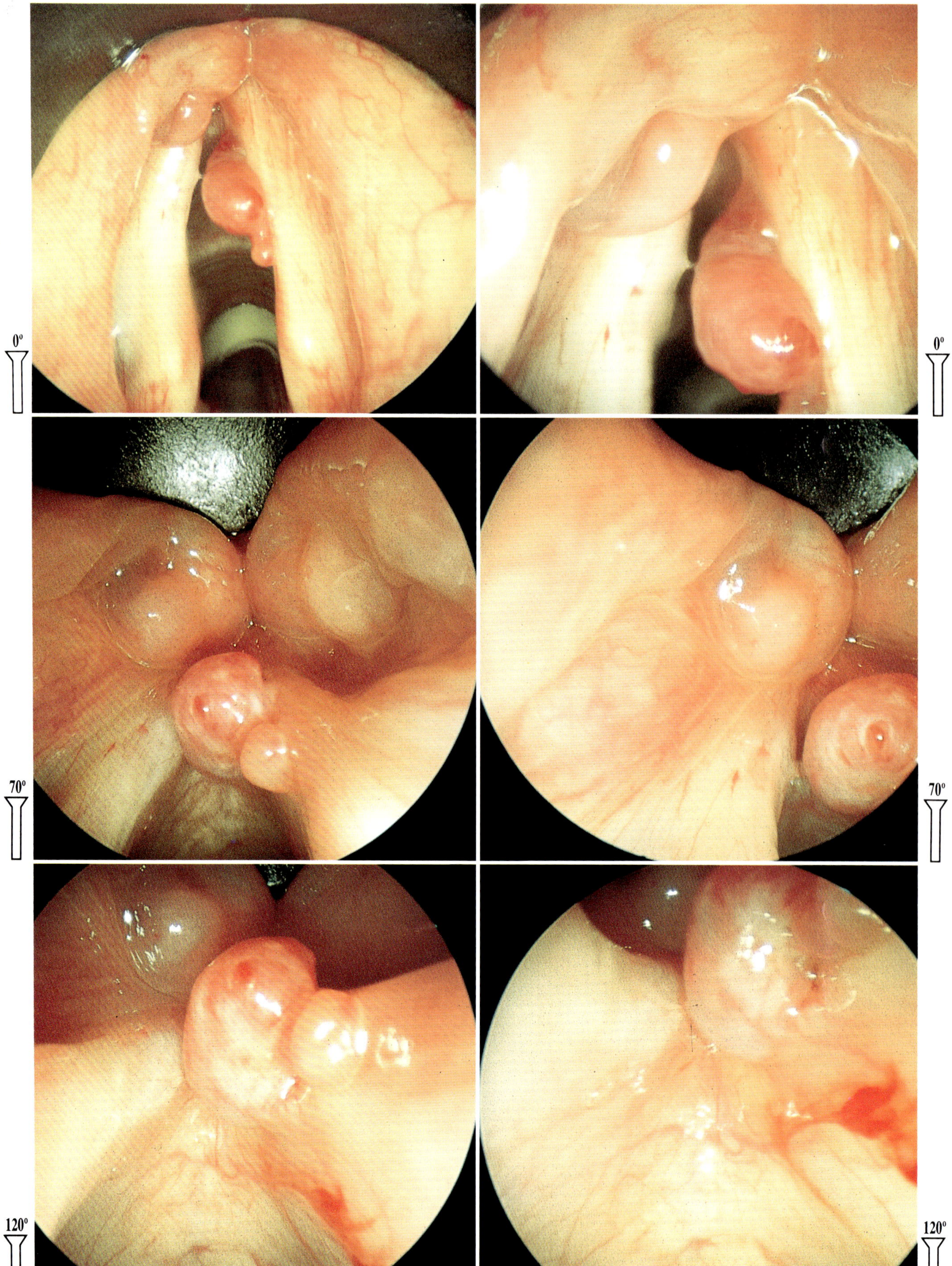
0°
0°
70°
70°
120°
120°

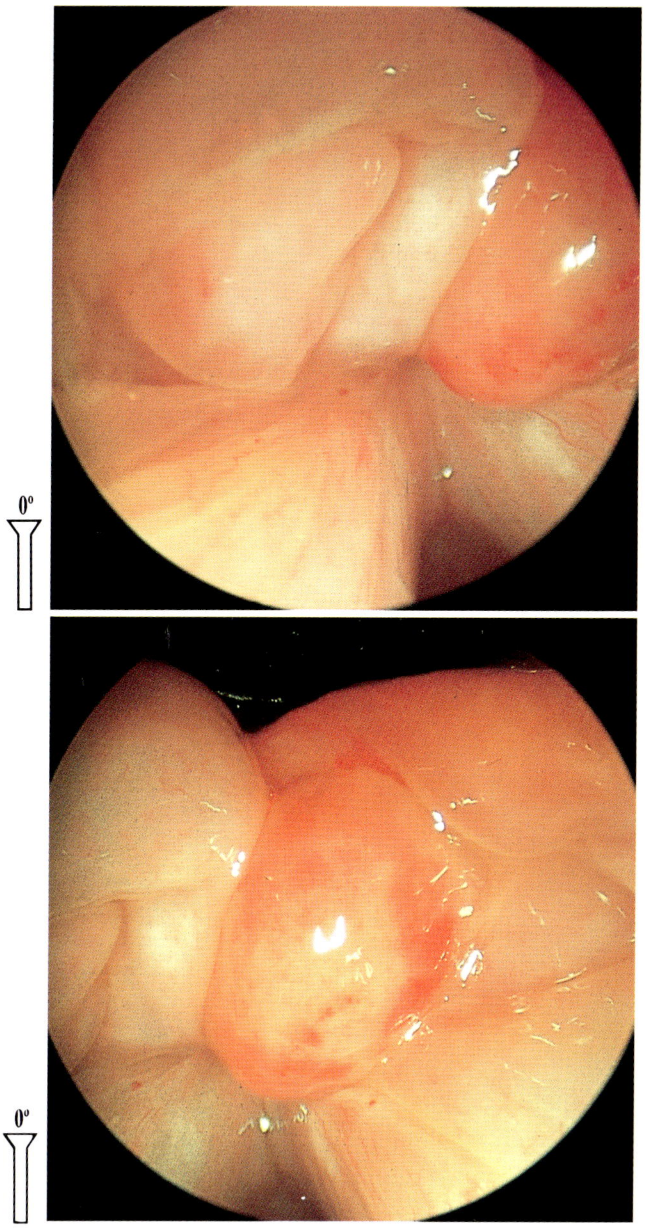

FIG. 26. This patient is a 45-year-old army officer. Mucosal eversion of both ventricles is observed with the 70° telescopes. The lesions seem to be at different stages of progression. The right side with its firm and hemorrhagic appearance is more advanced.

FIG. 25. This patient is a 53-year-old cigarette smoker and salesman. There is a large, multilobulated polyp at the anterior and middle part of the right vocal cord. As in other polyps described, keratinization is more significant at the inferior surface of the polypoid lesion. The large base of implantation is located at the free border and at the inferior surface of the vocal cord. Contralateral contact alterations are identified at the left vocal cord. Eversion of the mucosa of both Morgagni ventricles, accompanied by diffuse edema, is clearly observed with the 70° and 120° telescopes.

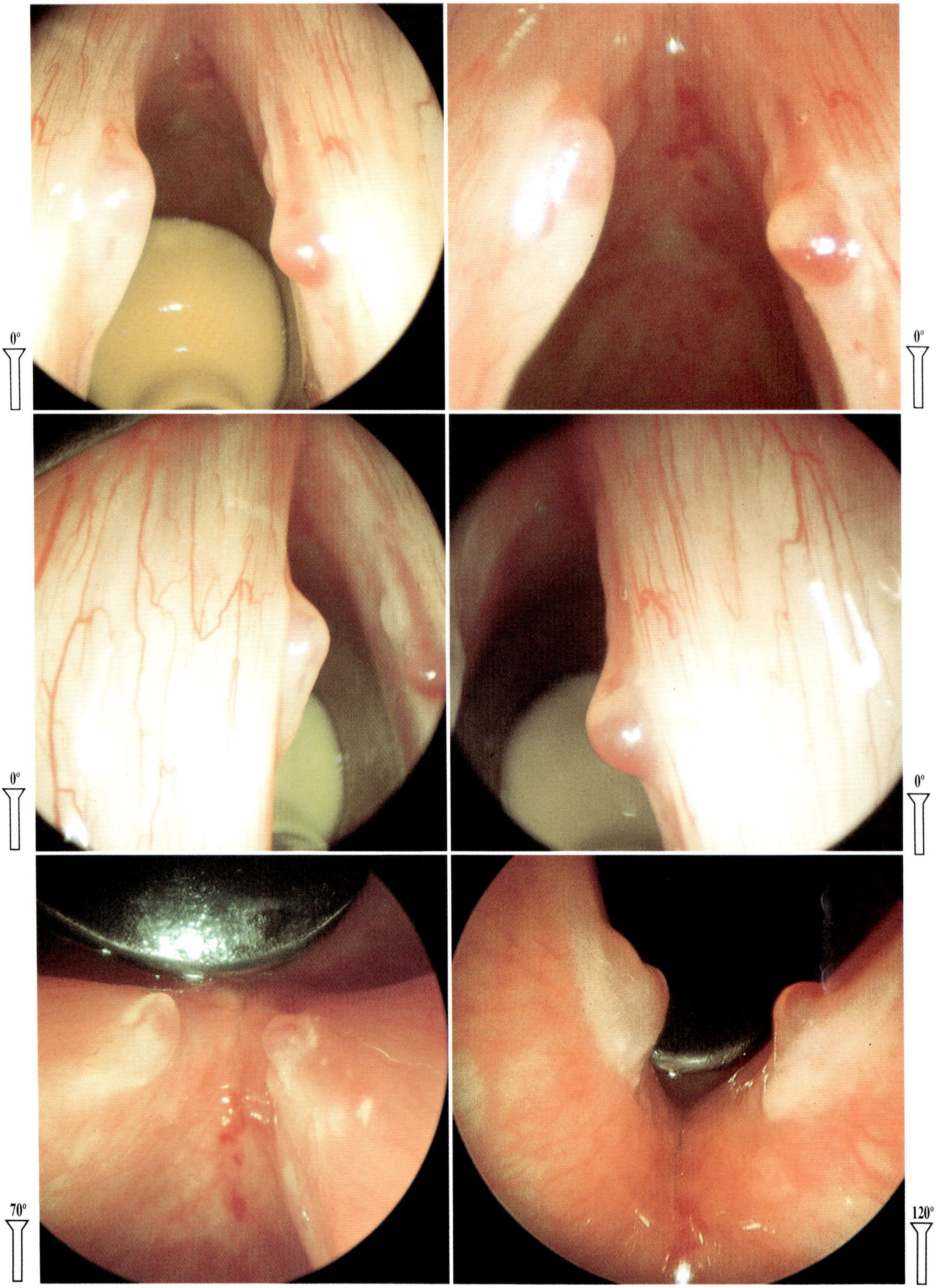
0°
0°
0°
0°
70°
120°

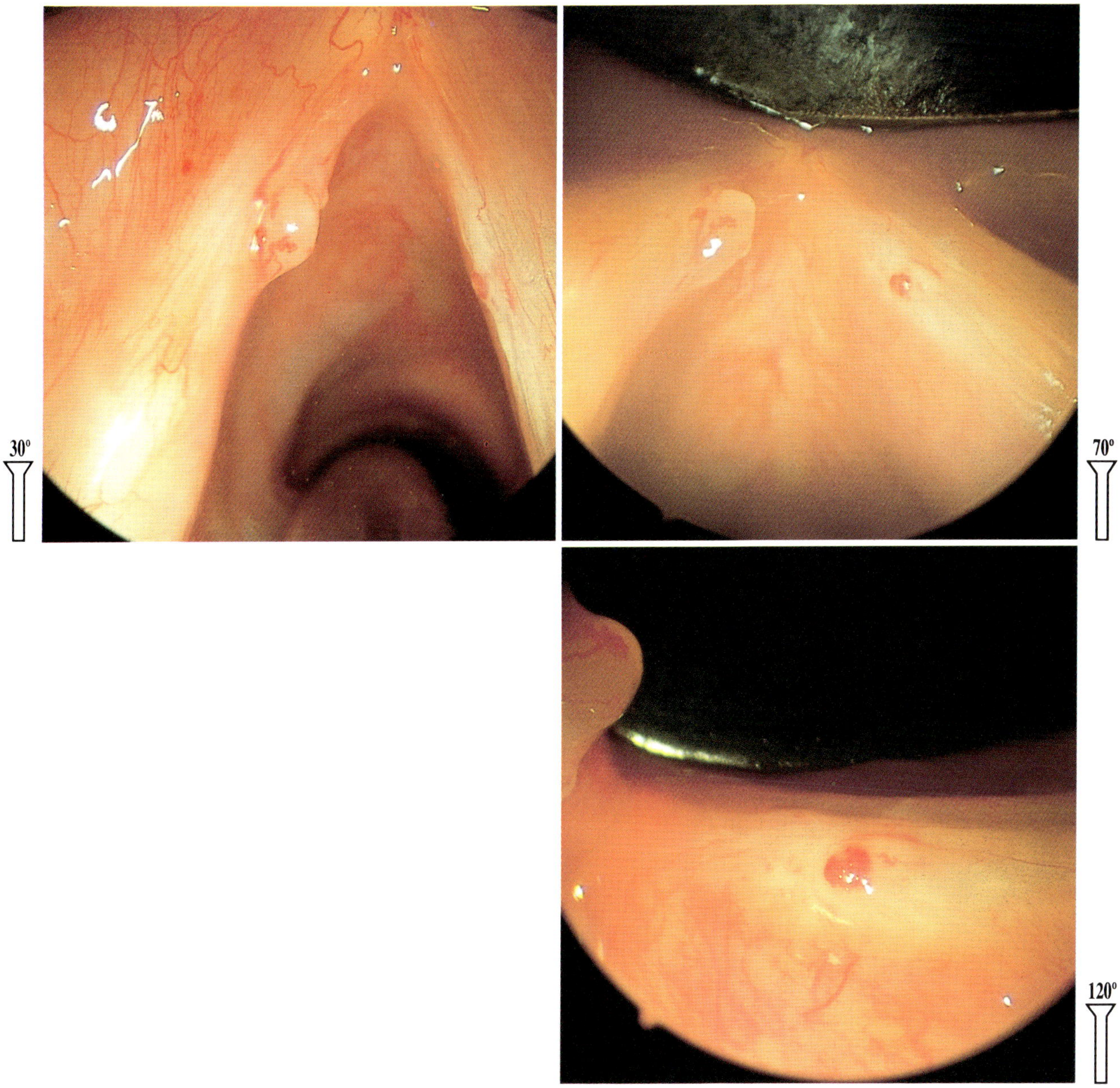

FIG. 28. This patient is a 35-year-old school teacher with vocal cord nodules in different stages of progression. Changes in vasculature are evident on both sides, with areas of keratosis at the free border and inferior surface.

FIG. 27. This 36-year-old man is a cigarette smoker and an agrarian engineer. There are bilateral vocal cord nodules with a translucent appearance at the middle third of the vocal cords. Significant areas of keratosis are identified at the inferior surface of the vocal cords using the 70° and 120° telescopes. Pathologic examination has confirmed the nodules

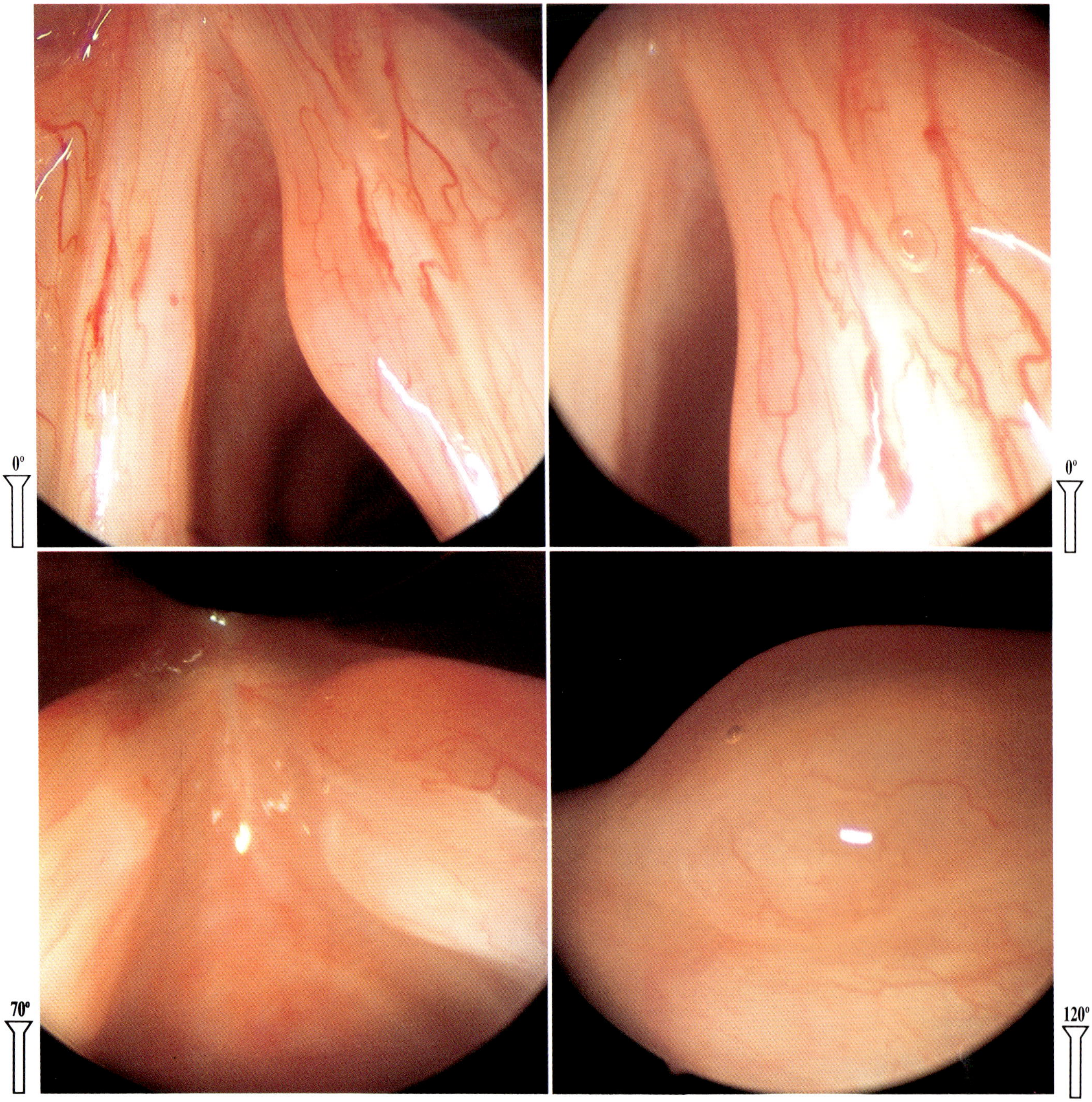

FIG. 29. This 43-year-old woman is a housekeeper. There is a cyst on the right vocal cord. Dilated vessels are at the superior surface of both vocal cords. Keratinization is present at the inferior surface of the lesion and at the contact area of the opposite cord.

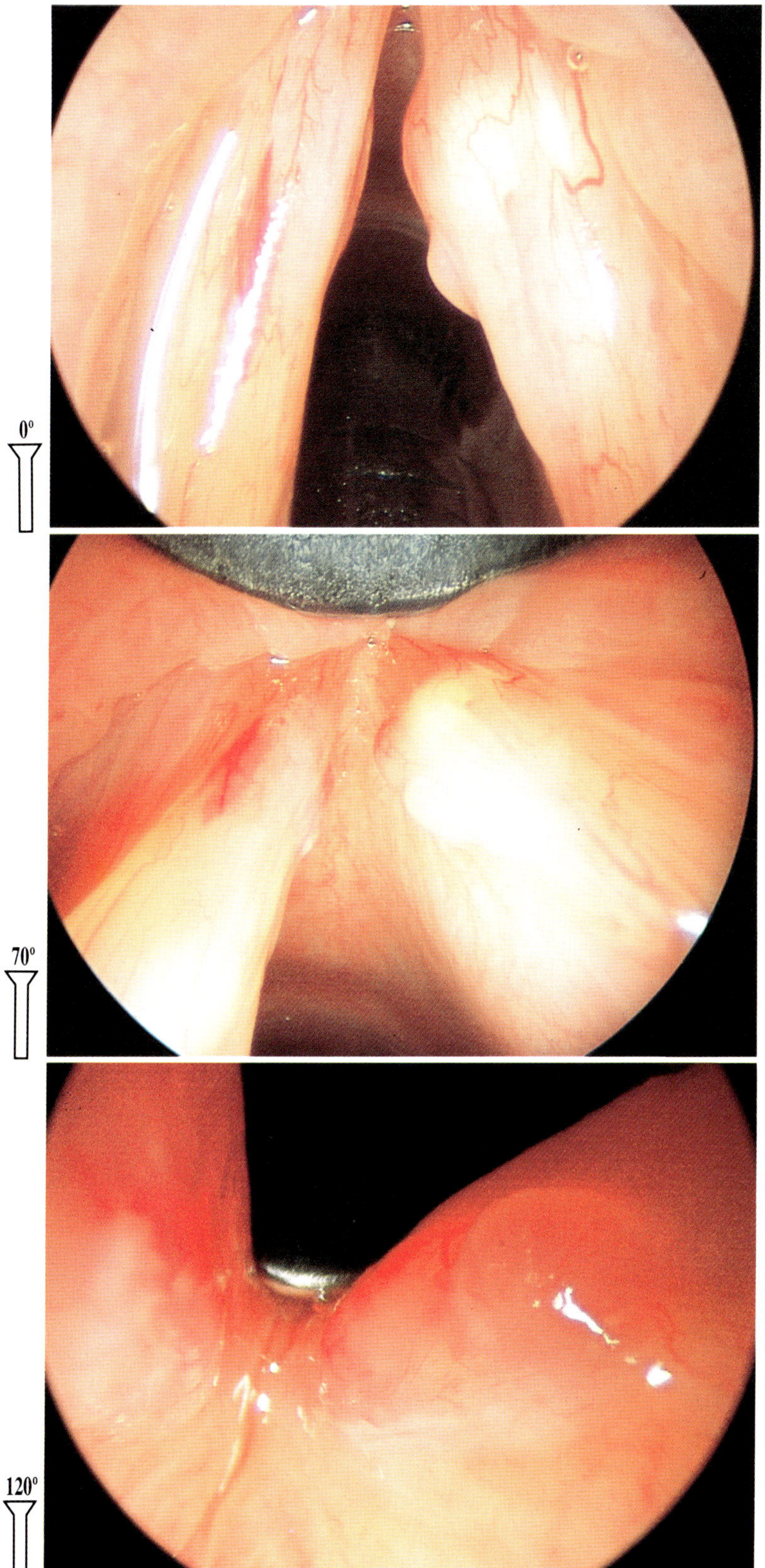

FIG. 30. This cyst at the vocal cord occurs in a 27-year-old pop-singer with a significant history of tobacco usage. Once again note the disturbed vascularity in both vocal cords.

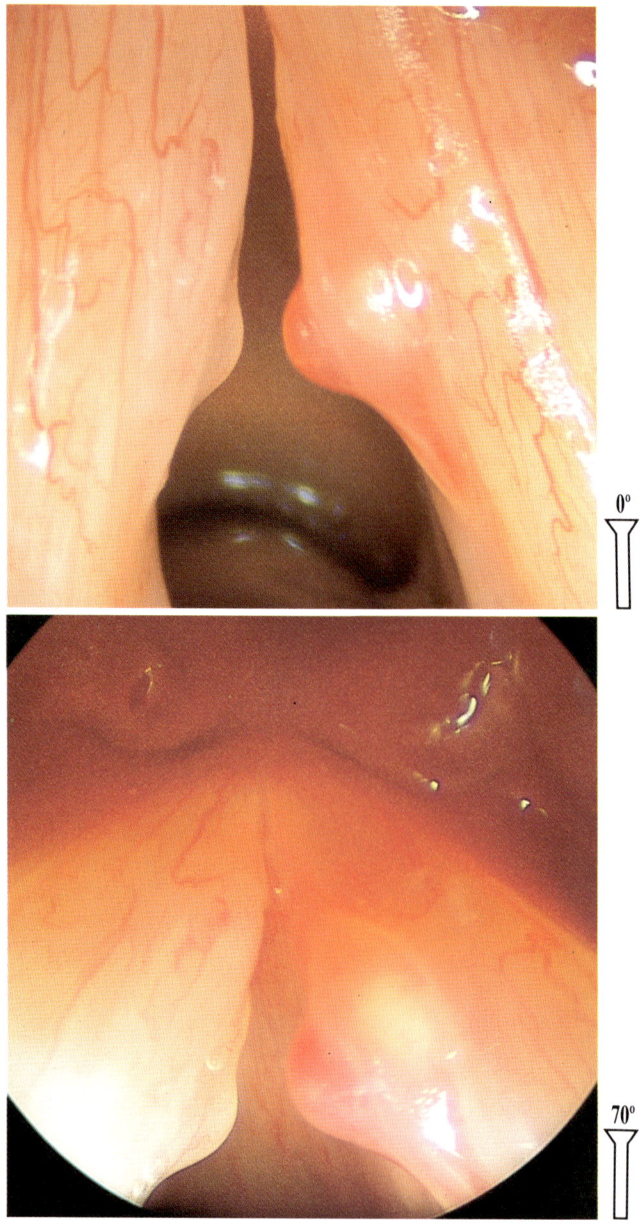

FIG. 31. This patient is a 37-year-old hairdresser with smoking habits. She has a submucosal right vocal cord cyst associated with bilateral polypoid lesions. The contour, color changes, and extent are clearly evaluated with the endoscopes.

FIG. 32. This patient is a 16-year-old boy. He has a large right glottosubglottic cyst that deforms the superior and inferior surfaces of the vocal cord and the subglottis. CT and MRI confirm the cystic nature of the lesion.

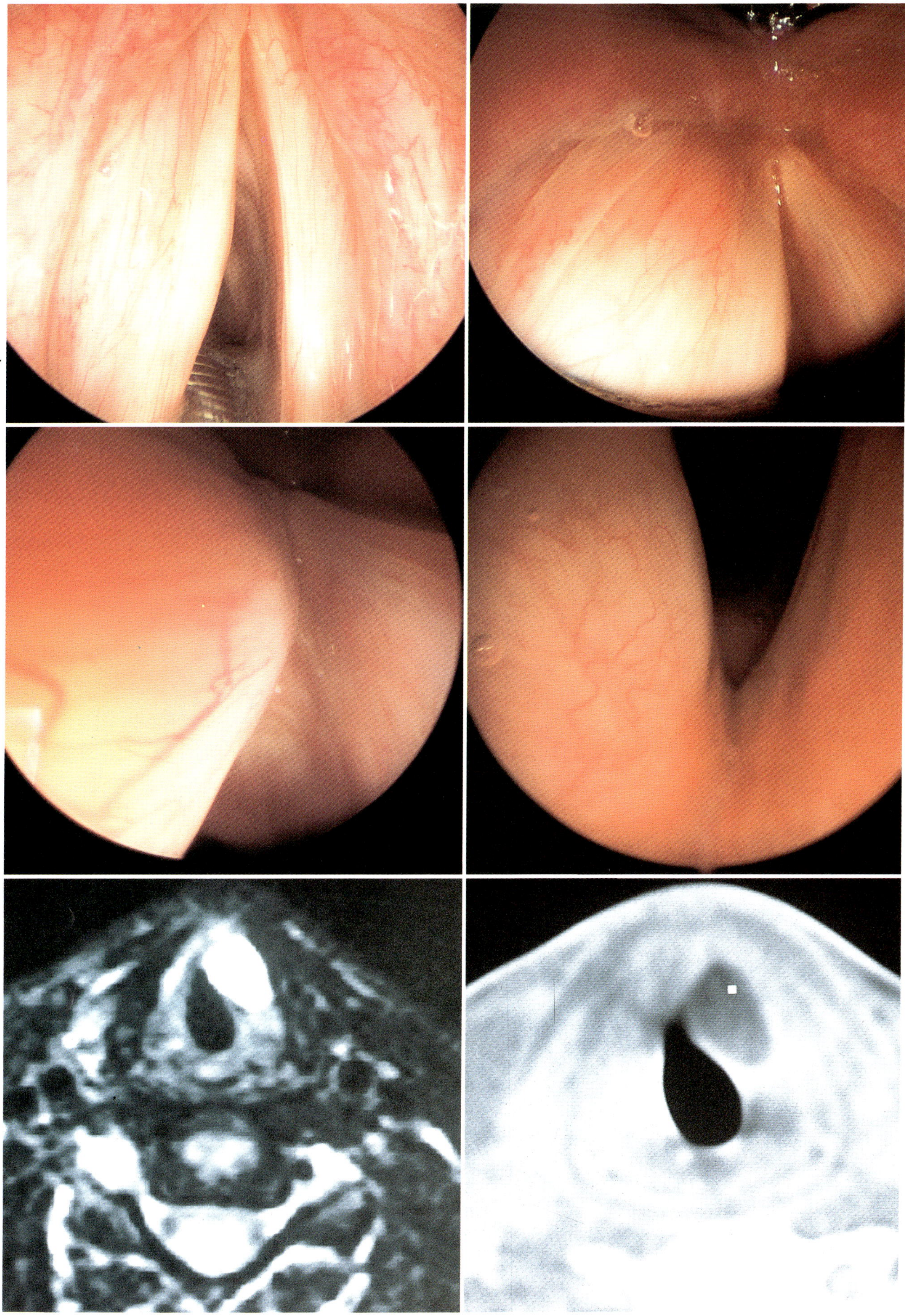

0°

70°

70°

120°

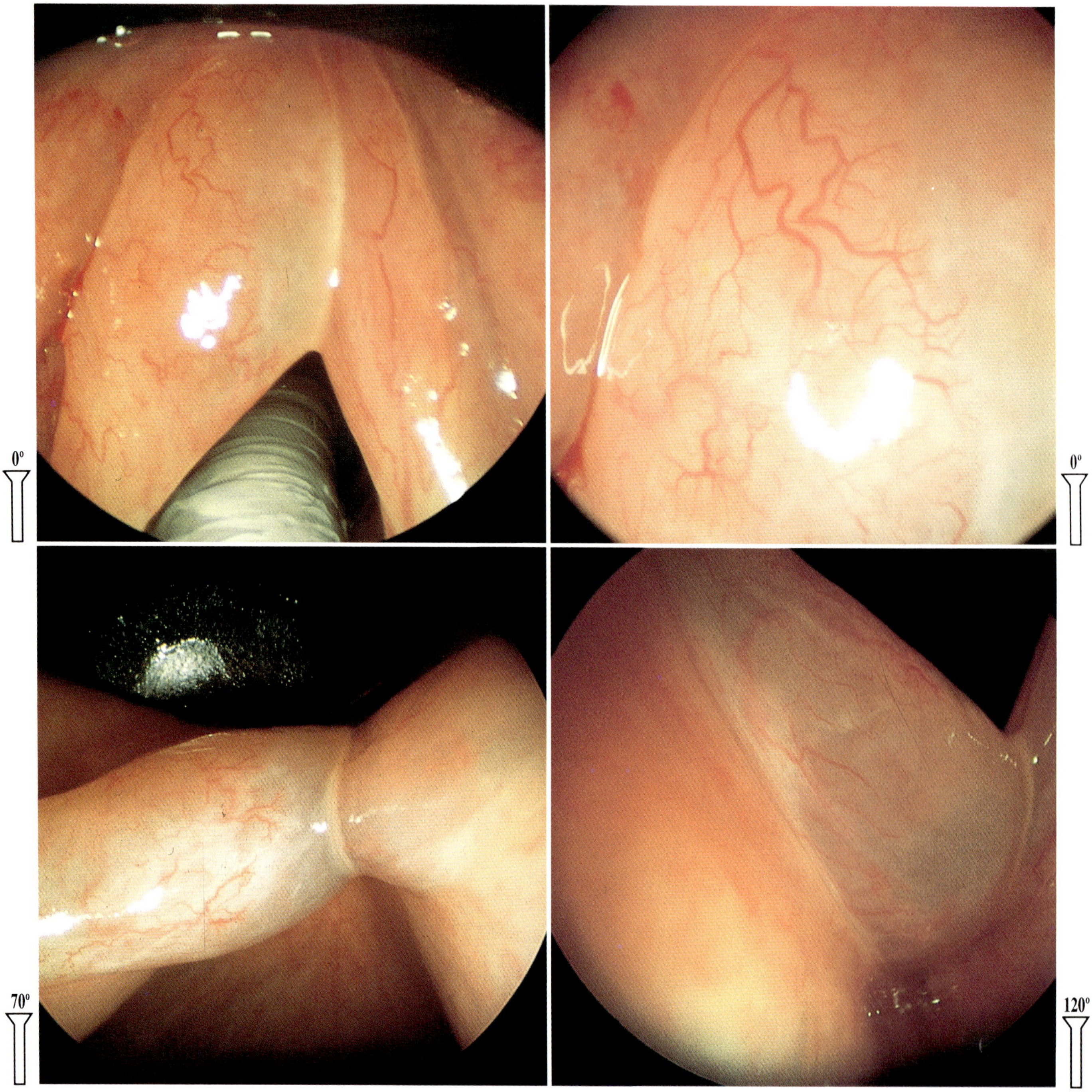

FIG. 33. This 61-year-old man is a cigarette smoker and an agrarian engineer with chronic sinusitis. He has bilateral Reinke's edema that is more pronounced at the left vocal cord. The subepithelial edema stretches the blood vessels of the superior surface. Diffuse keratosis is more significant in the contact areas between the vocal cords. With the 120° endoscope, the inferior limit of Reinke's edema (inferior linea arcuata) can be identified.

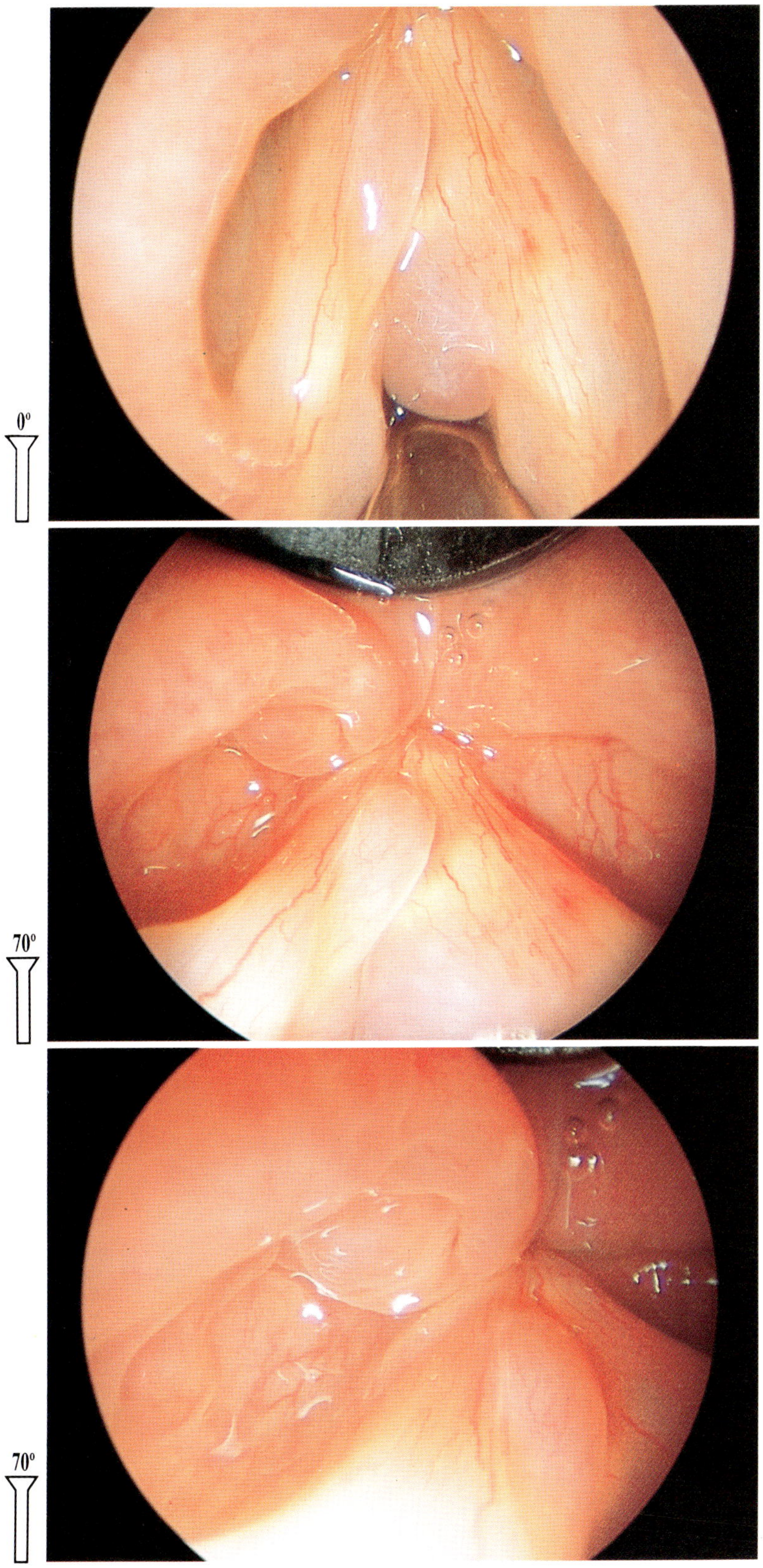

FIG. 34. This patient is a 44-year-old policeman with smoking habits. The mucosa appears loose and edematous. The edema is more pronounced on the right side and has the appearance of a broad based polypoid lesion. Also, note the prolapse of the anterior left ventricular mucosa.

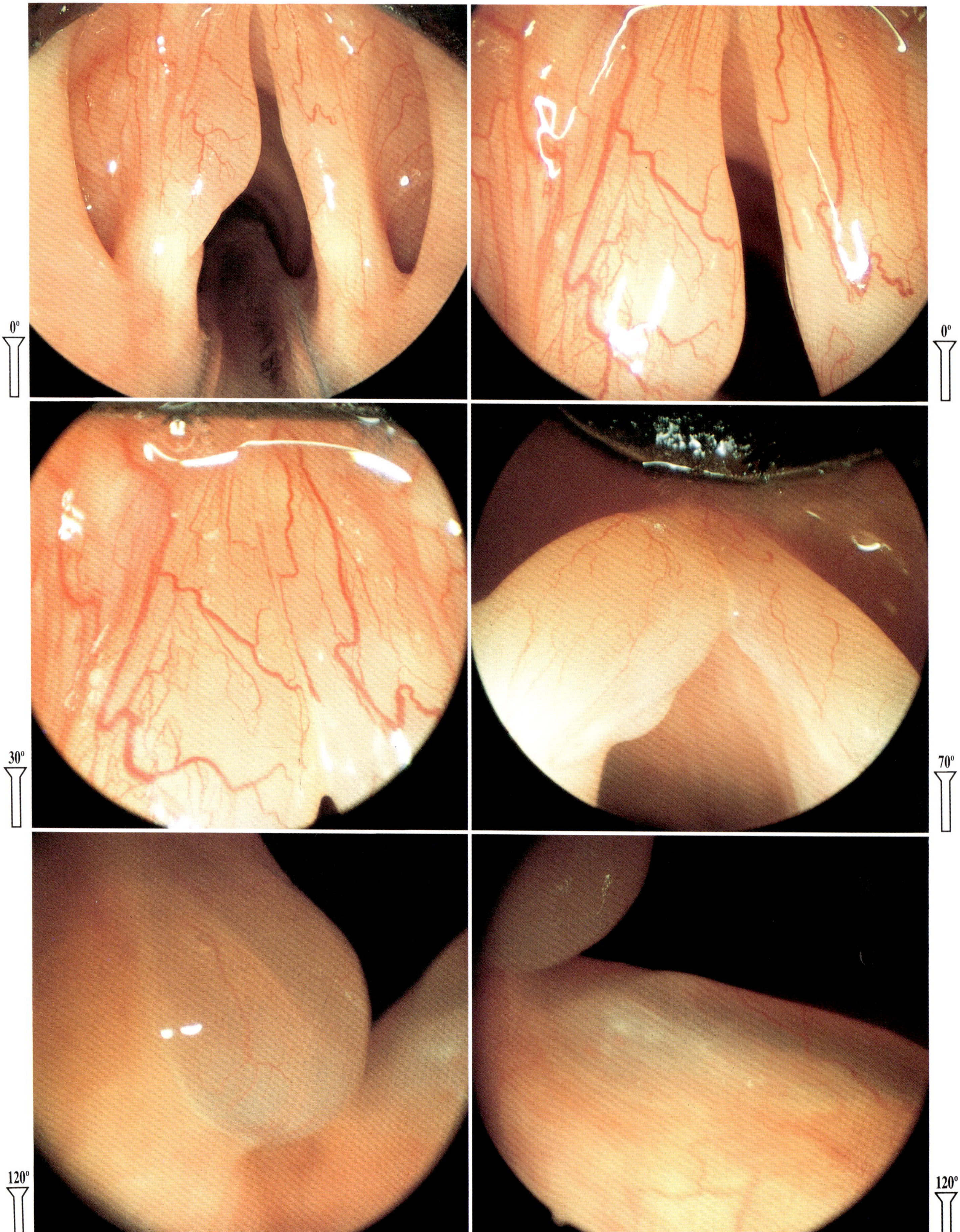
0°
0°
30°
70°
120°
120°

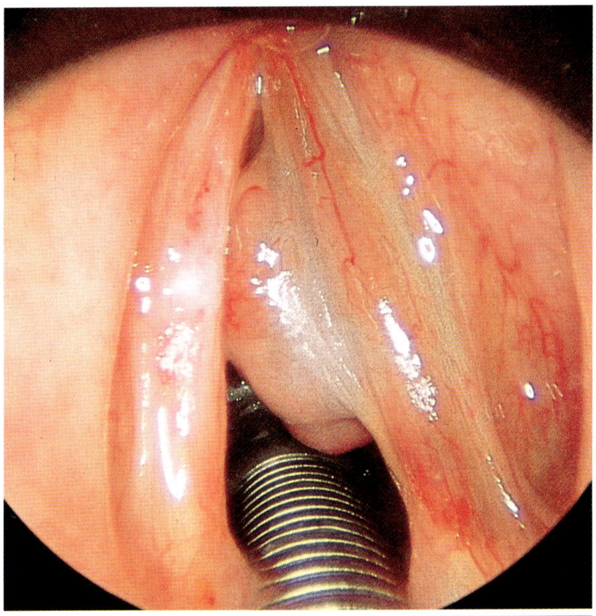

0°

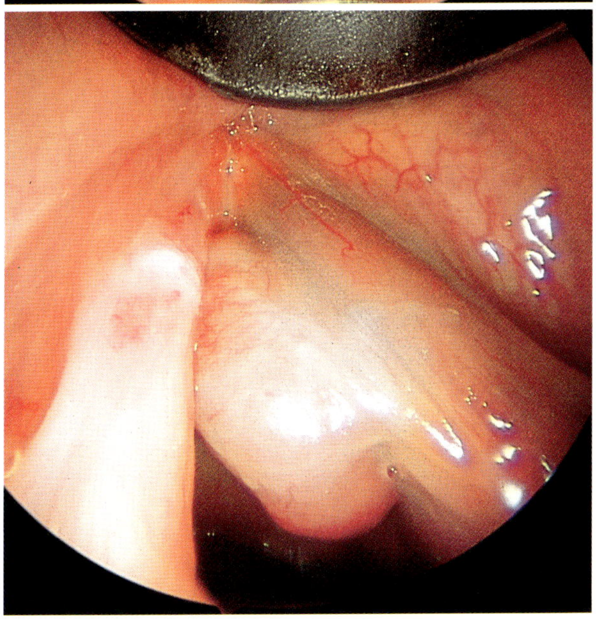

70°

FIG. 36. This is a 46-year-old salesman with smoking habits. There is a polypoid formation associated with diffuse edema along the right vocal cord. Keratosis and vascular changes are also noted along the left vocal cord.

FIG. 35. This 37-year-old nurse is a cigarette smoker. Early-stage bilateral Reinke's edema is more pronounced on the left side. The blood vessels are stretched by the accumulated fluid. At the inferior surface of the lesions, slight signs of keratosis are visible. On the left side, the inferior linea arcuata limits the Reinke's edema.

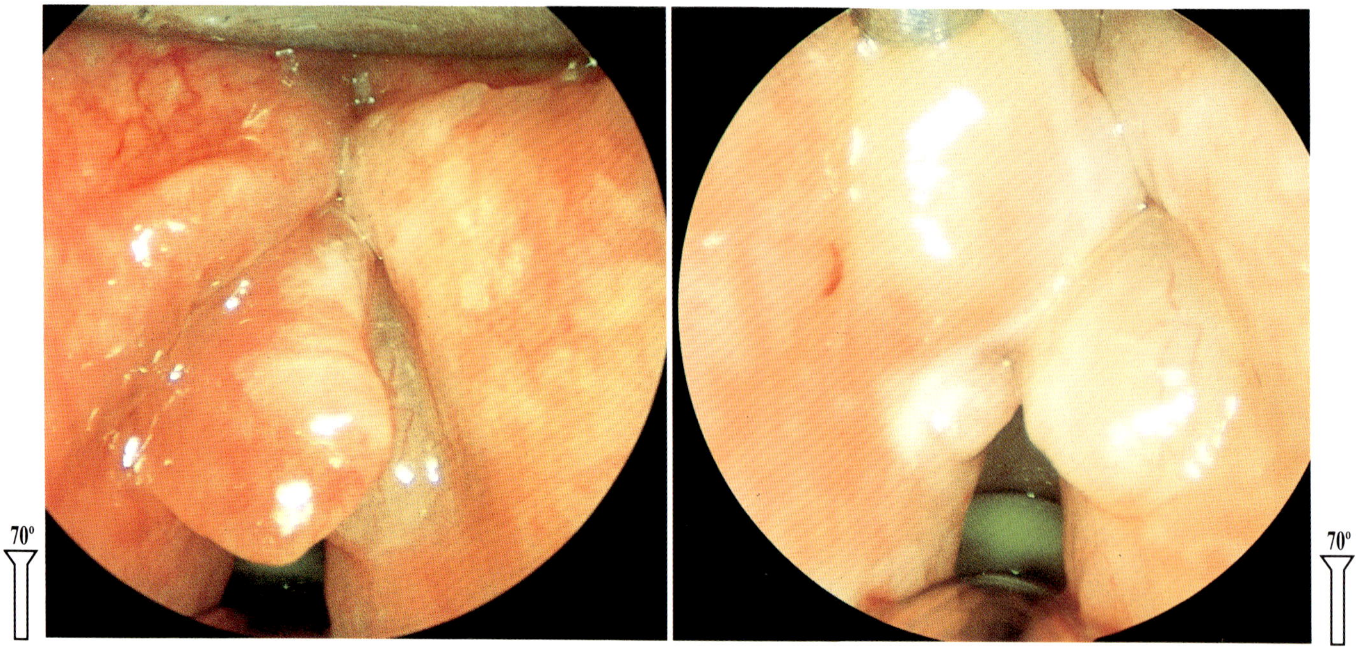

FIG. 37. This 61-year-old man is a cigarette smoker and a bus driver. He has advanced bilateral Reinke's edema. Keratotic areas are evident. The lesion of the left side is displaced by the suction tube. Diffuse inflammatory signs are also present at the false cords.

The definition of the anterior and posterior limits of a polyp that are not always evident when observed through the microscope are well established with the telescopes, allowing the identification of the transition between the polyp and the normal mucosa.

Assessment of the glottis with 70° and 120° endoscopes identifies significant features of the mucosa of the inferior surface and the free border of the vocal cord, and of the vasculature in phonation disorders.

REMS also permits a much better view of the opposite vocal cord. Areas of edema, hyperplasia, queratosis, and depressions of the free border can be observed when examining the primary lesion; these areas are normally poorly visualized or possibly missed by single microscopic evaluation.

Concerning nodules, the use of endoscopes provides a much more detailed evaluation. Besides form, relief, and surface characteristics, it is possible to observe the inferior surface of the nodule and of the vocal cord.

Looking at the nodule from below and from behind and observing all the alterations of the mucosa, the understanding of its physiopathology and its developmental stage is improved.

The notion of trauma is evidenced by the symmetric queratotic and edematous areas at the inferior surface of both vocal cords.

This precise assessment provides a better therapeutic approach and rigid endoscopic video images can be shared between surgeons and speech pathologists.

Cysts that have already benefited from stroboscopy become more evident with REMS—site, dimensions and relief.

The mucosal vessels are identified and the surgical approach is well established.

The differential diagnosis of early stages of polyps, nodules, and cysts can also be improved with the detailed evaluation through the telescopes.

In cases with benign pathology, the coexistence of additional pathology other than that viewed by microlaryngoscopy is not uncommon, as it happens with small leukoplakias present in cases of nodules and polyps.

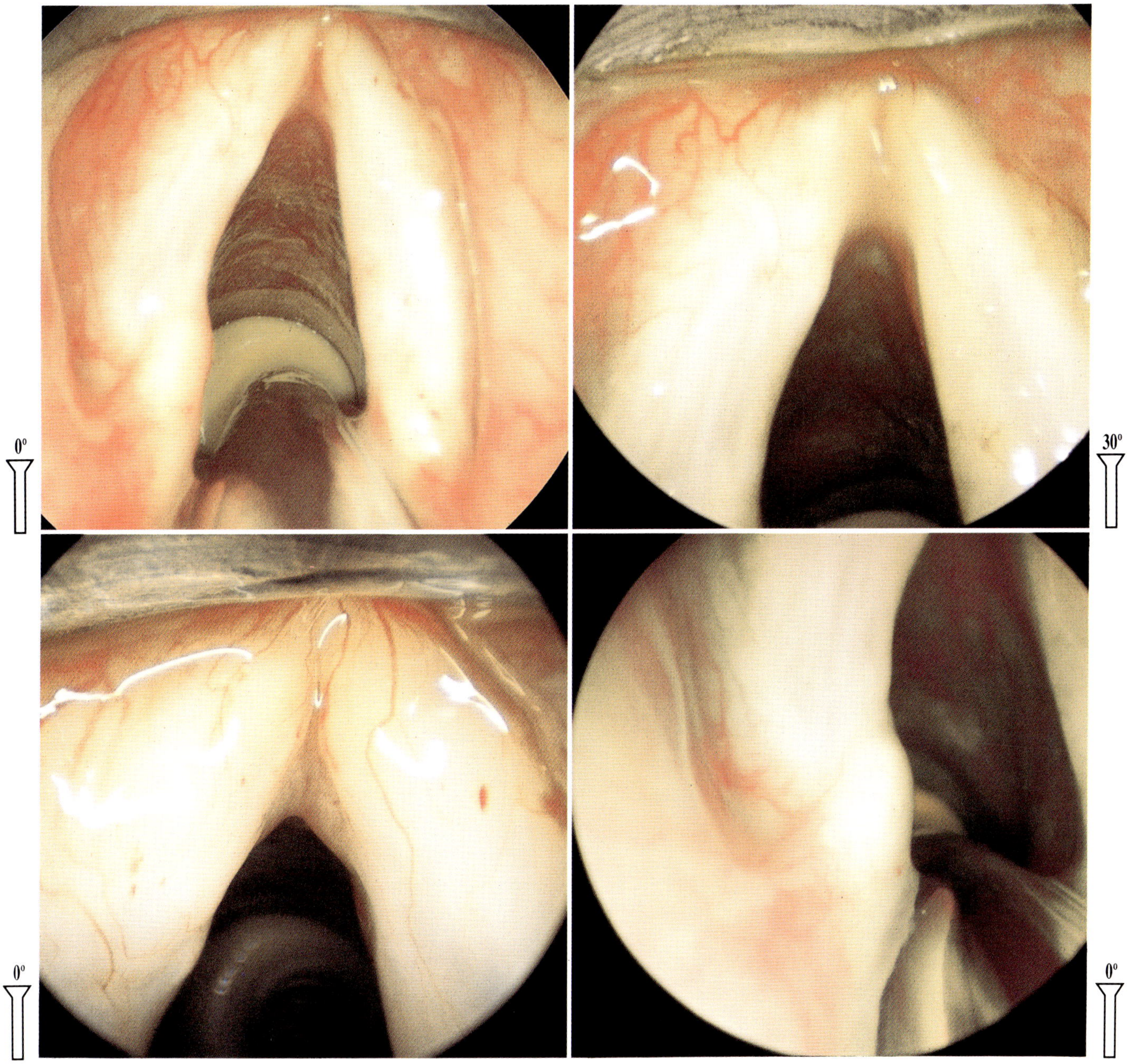

FIG. 38. This 41-year-old woman is a post office worker. She has vocal cord atrophy after having had bilateral removal of Reinke's edema performed 8 years before. A prominent vocal process is evident on the left side.

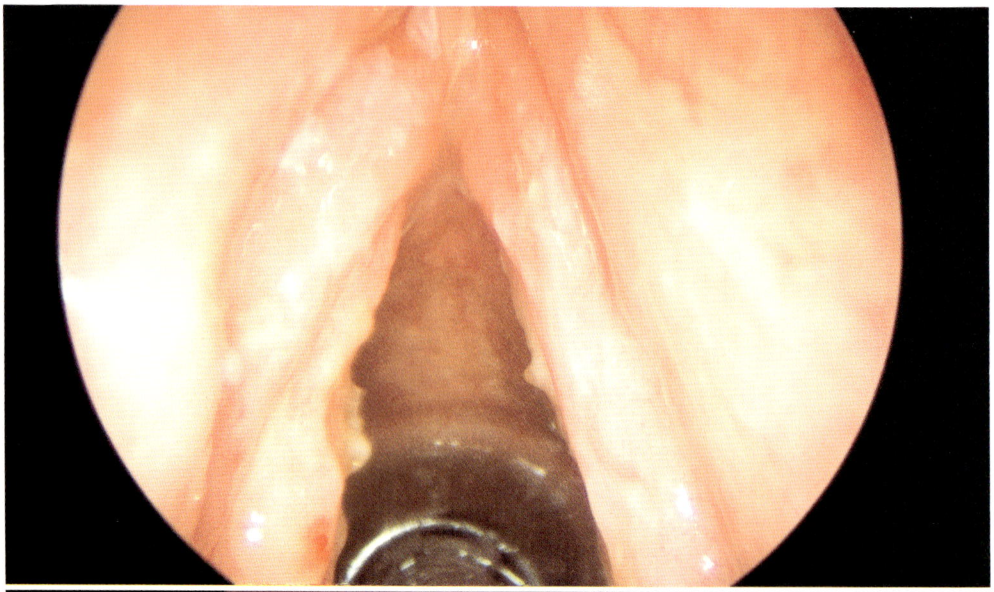

0°

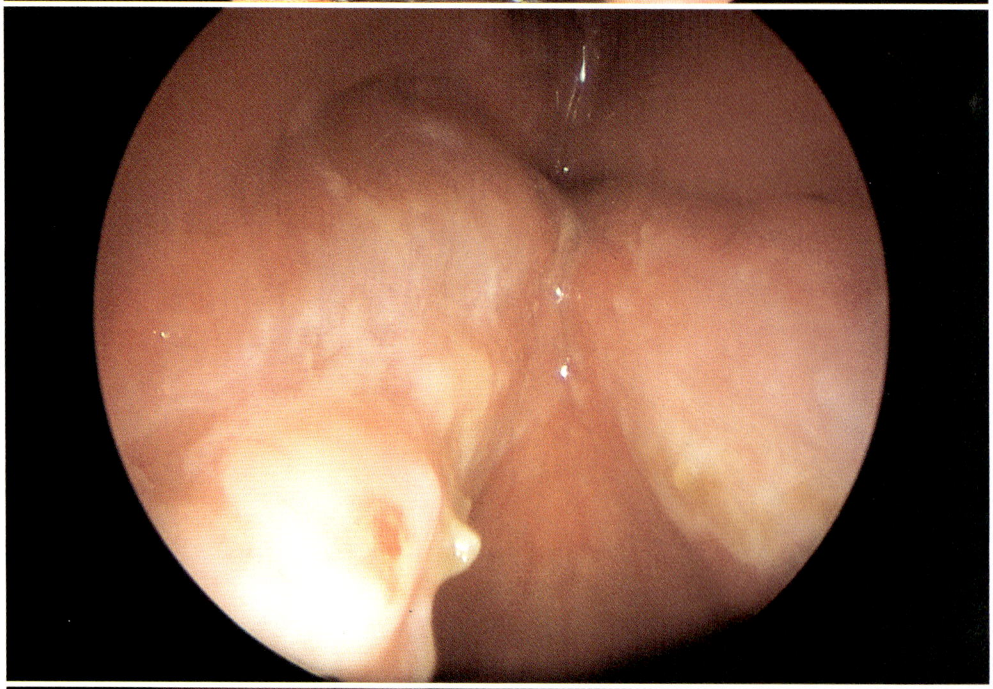

70°

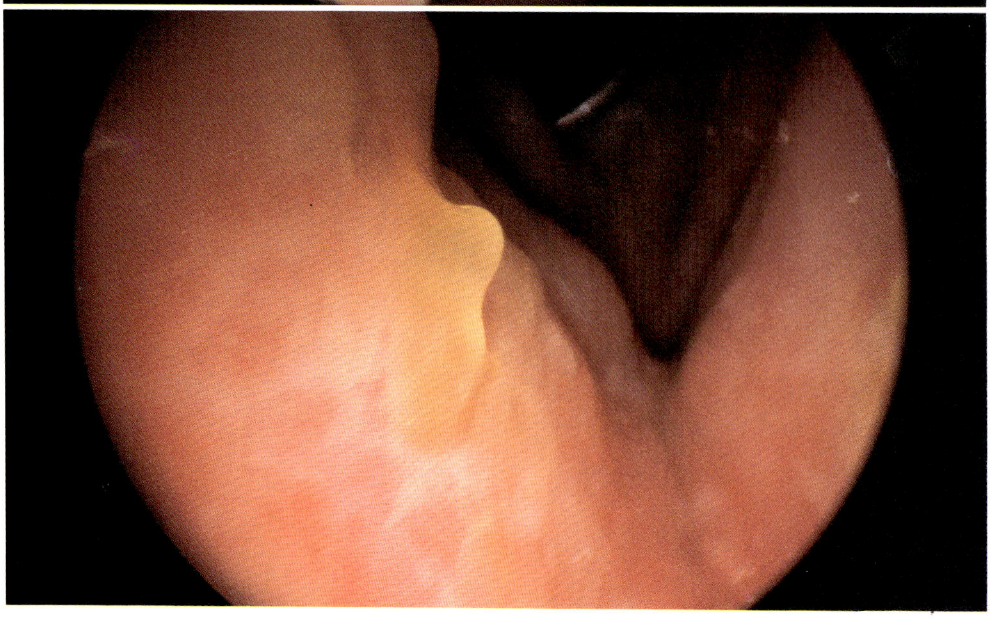

120°

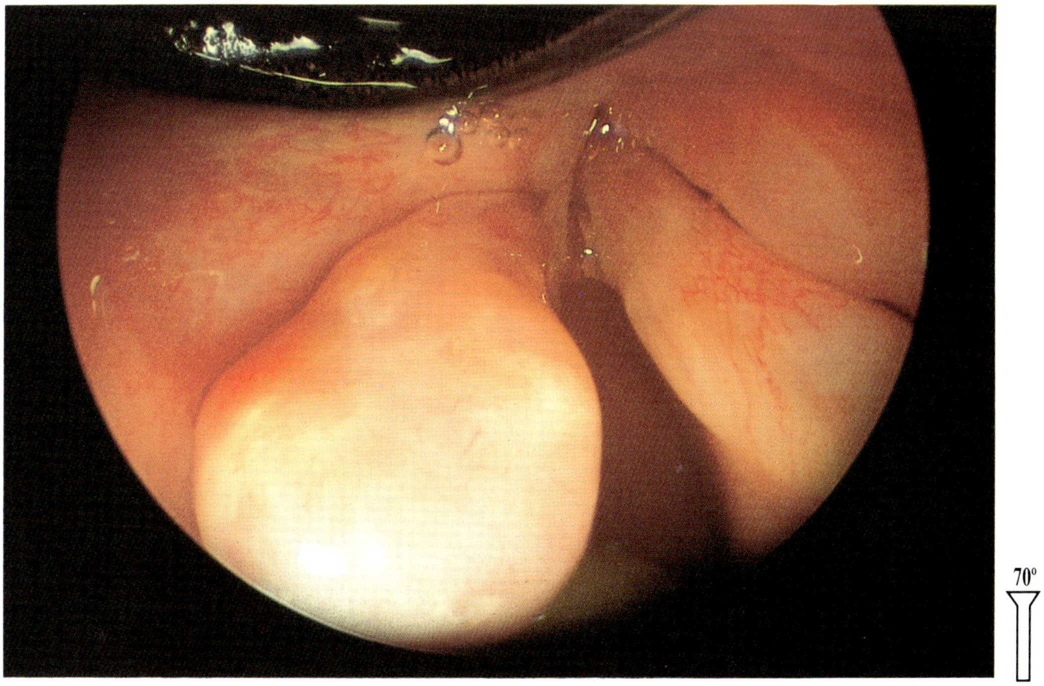

FIG. 40. Chronic laryngitis and Reinke's edema, particularly evident along the left side, are seen in this 53-year-old smoker.

FIG. 39. This 47-year-old man is a cigarette smoker with chronic sinusitis. He has chronic hyperplastic laryngitis. There are diffuse and intense signs of inflammation throughout the larynx.

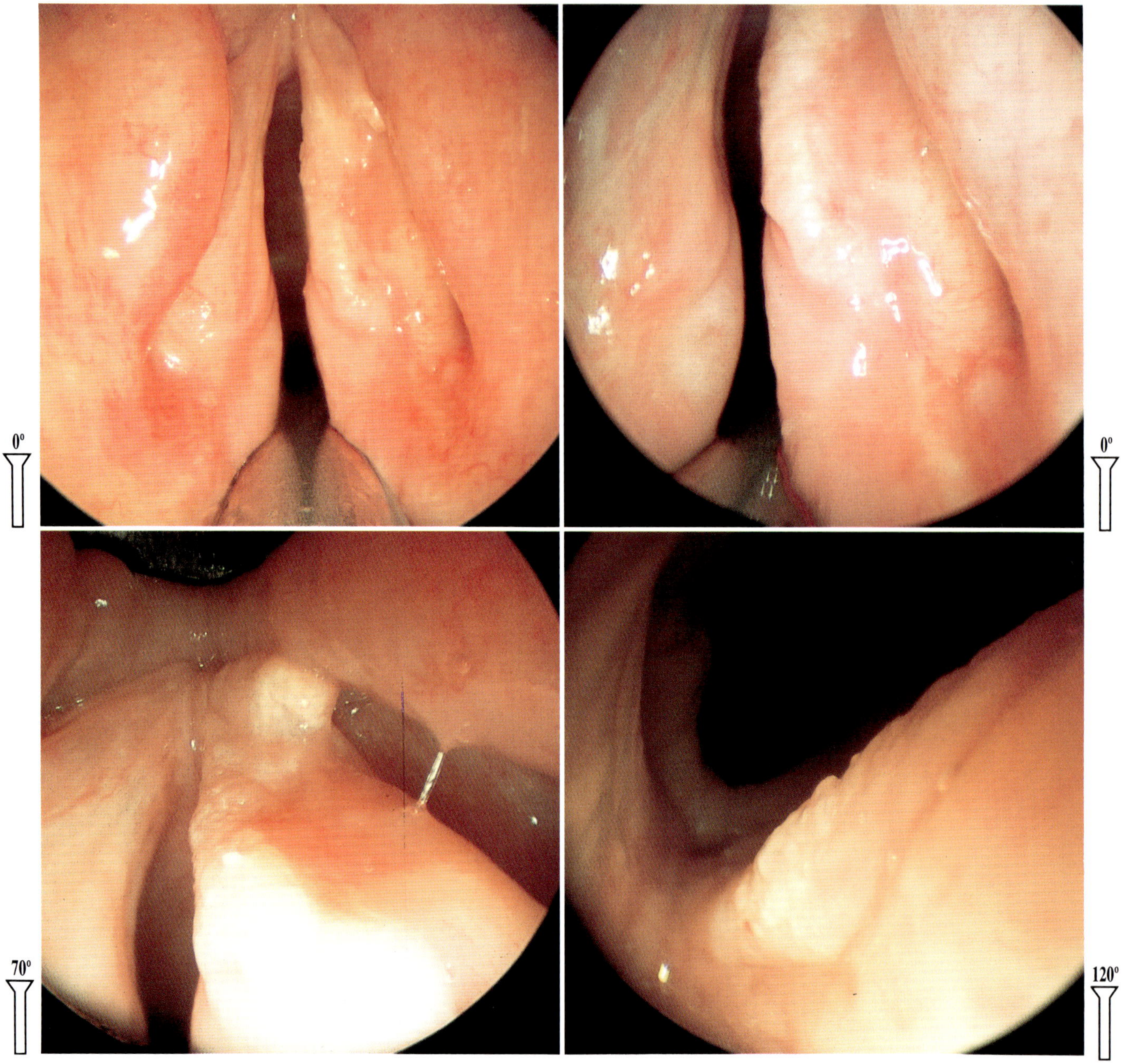

FIG. 41. This 55-year-old man is a cigarette smoker and a textile worker. He has chronic hyperplastic laryngitis. The relief of the lesion is particularly evident with the 70° endoscope.

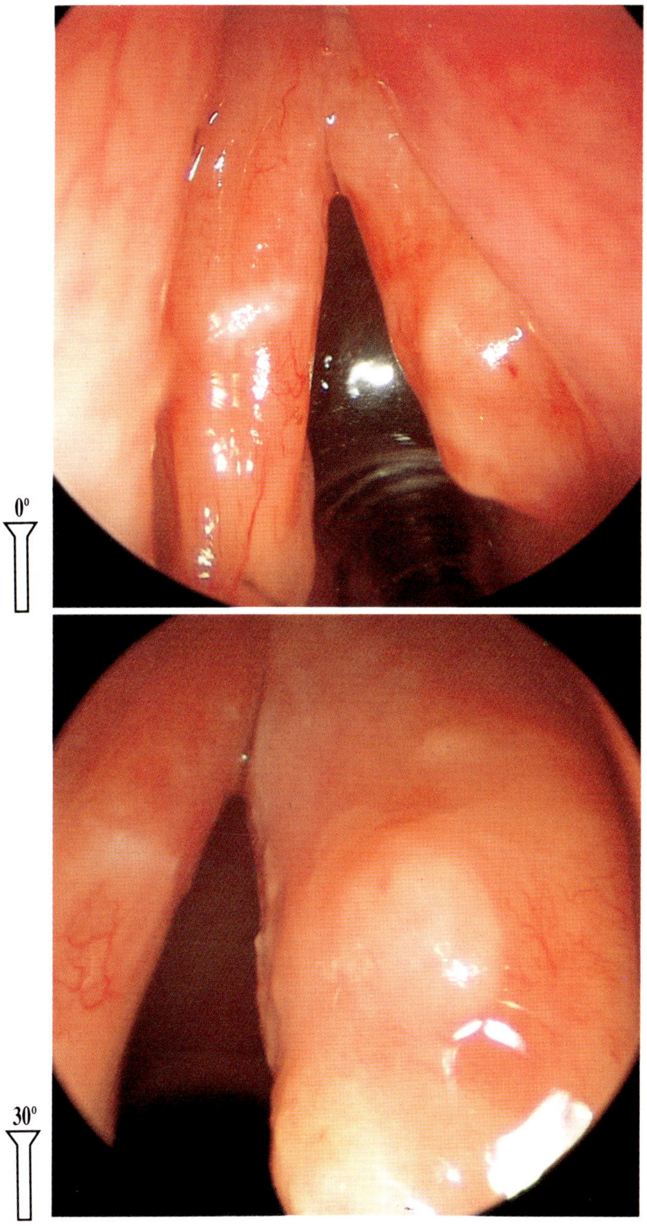

FIG. 42. Chronic inflammation of both vocal cords is seen in this 45-year-old non-smoking patient. History was also remarkable for a recent move from Africa, and telescopes allowed documentation of the characteristics of this lesion, which was subsequently shown to be Histoplasmosis.

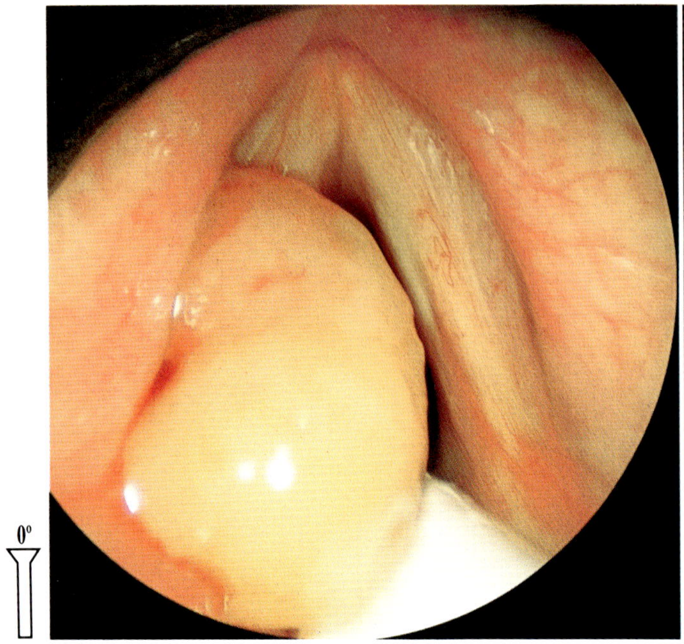

FIG. 43. This 64-year-old man is a cigarette smoker and a public officer. He has contact granuloma of the arytenoid region associated with gastroesophageal reflux.

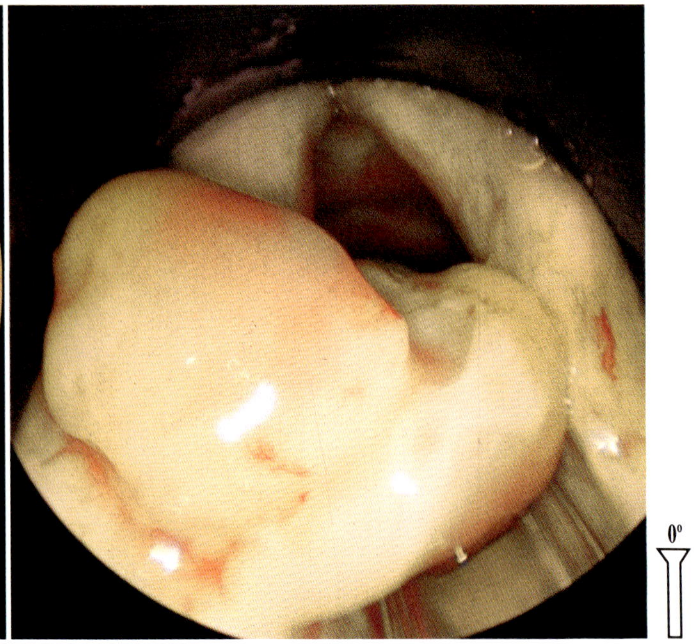

FIG. 44. This 40-year-old man is a bank employee. He has contact granuloma of the arytenoid region associated with gastroesophageal reflux.

Assessment of benign lesions influences phonosurgery techniques. In polyps, the improved observation allowed by REMS, including the base of the lesion, the inferior surface of the vocal cord, and the vascular pedicles, provides information that can influence subsequent instrumental or CO_2 laser microsurgery. Medial traction of the polyp, displacing it from the vocal cord ligament, may cause unnecessary sacrifice of the mucosa of the inferior surface of the vocal cord, compromising phonation.

It is interesting to note that in microlaryngeal surgery of vocal polyps, concern is usually focused on the superior surface of the vocal cords, although polyps originate from the mucosa of the inferior surface of the vocal cords as becomes evident after REMS evaluation. In fact, the base and the main vascular pedicle of the polyp are situated at the inferior surface, which is important when considering phonosurgery technique. Refinement of the surgical technique and new instruments will certainly occur following this multiperspective and highly-detailed assessment of benign lesions.

Surgery through the microscope has the advantage of the simultaneous use of both hands. In some cases, surgical gestures performed through the microscope have been monitored through one of the angled endoscopes coupled with a video camera. Microlaryngeal surgery will evolve towards what happened in endoscopic nasal surgery in which microscope and endoscopes are used in articulation, complementing each other.

In Reinke's edema, the telescopes allowed to establish its limits—anterior, posterior, laterally and also inferiorly. If the relationships between the floor of the ventricle, the anterior commissure, and the vocal process are important to define the surgical technique, REMS have permitted to look from the subglottis to the inferior surface of the vocal cord and to observe the inferior limit of Reinke's edema.

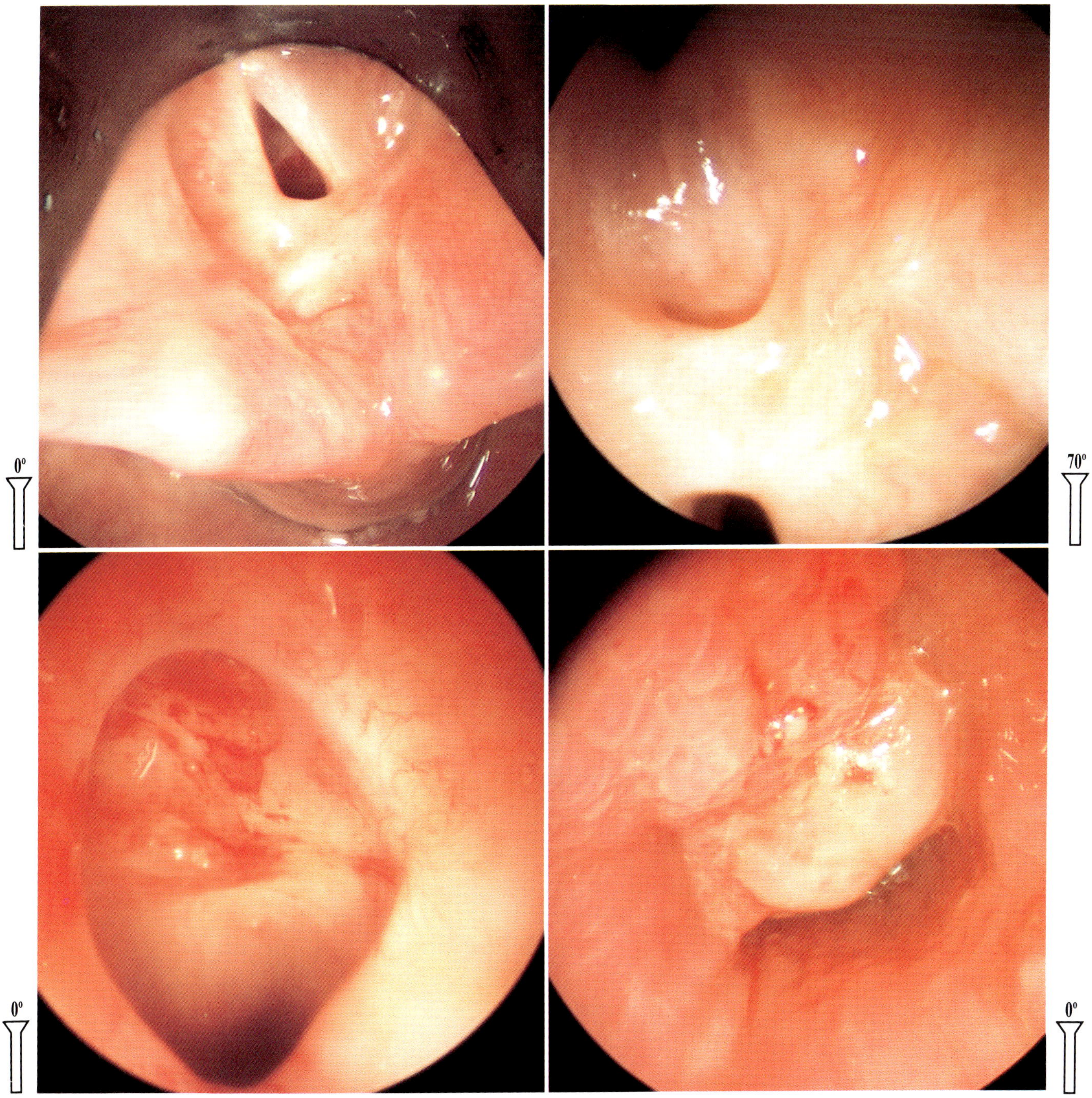

FIG. 45. This 9-year-old patient has sequelae of intubation. Three separate lesions compromising the airway at different levels can be identified: a synechia of the posterior commissure, a thin stenotic ring at the subglottis, and a granuloma above the tracheotomy.

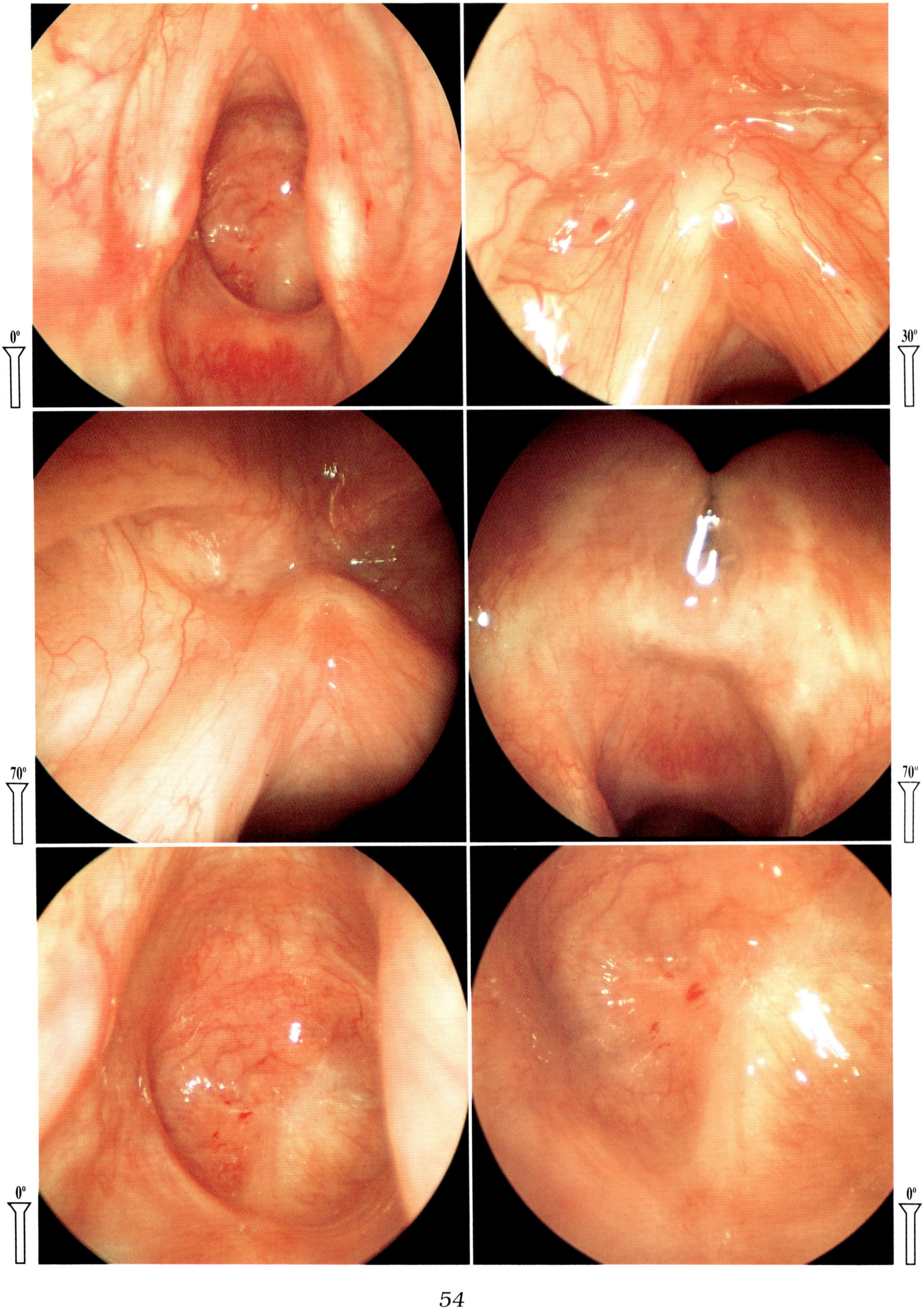
0°
30°
70°
70°
0°
0°

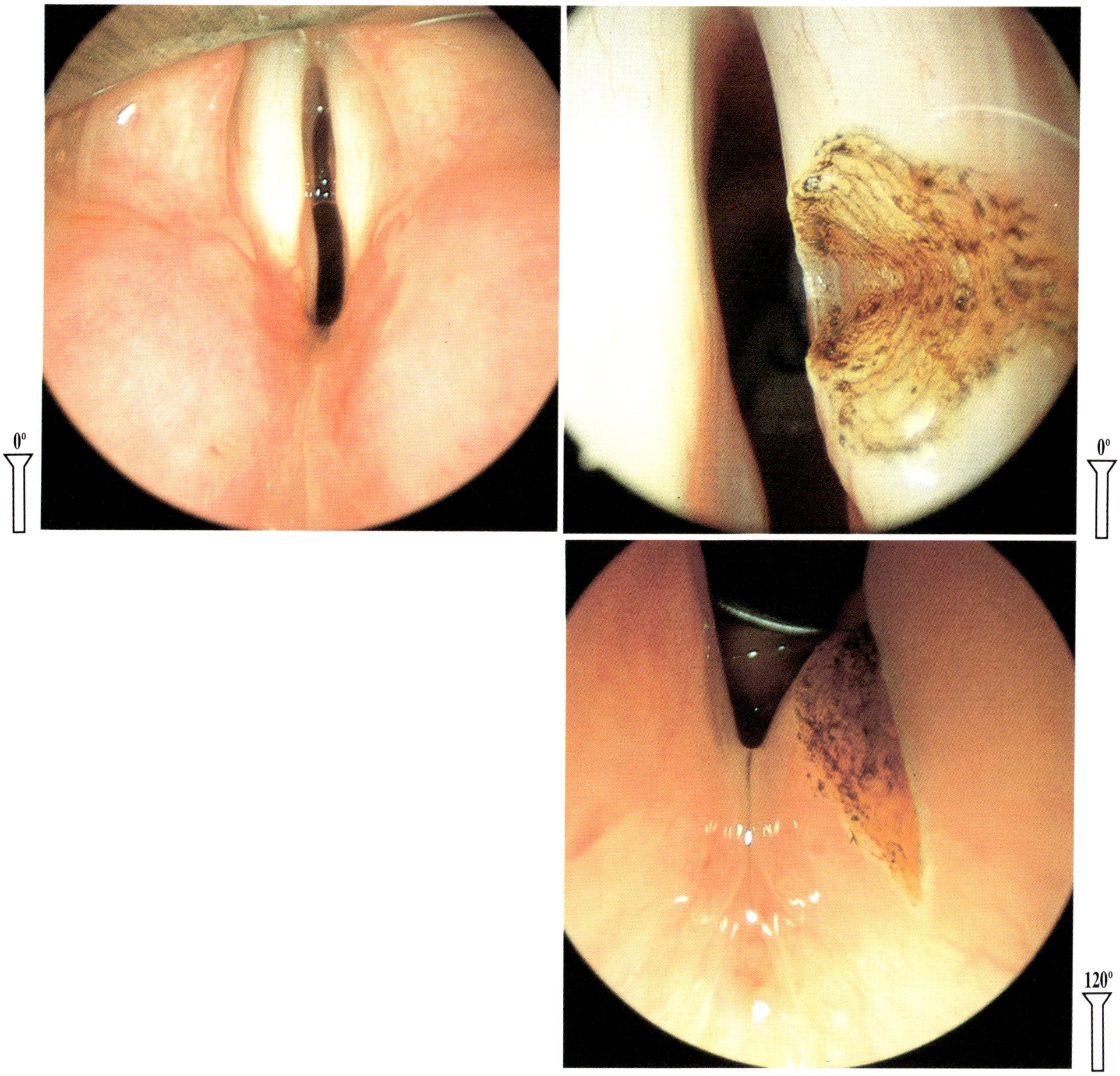

FIG. 47. This 55-year-old woman has bilateral vocal cord paralysis, status post total thyroidectomy. Intraoperative telescopic images during CO_2 laser posterior cordotomy allow a controlled surgical technique.

FIG. 46. This 19-year-old man has a postintubation sequela. Complete subglottic stenosis is observed with REMS.

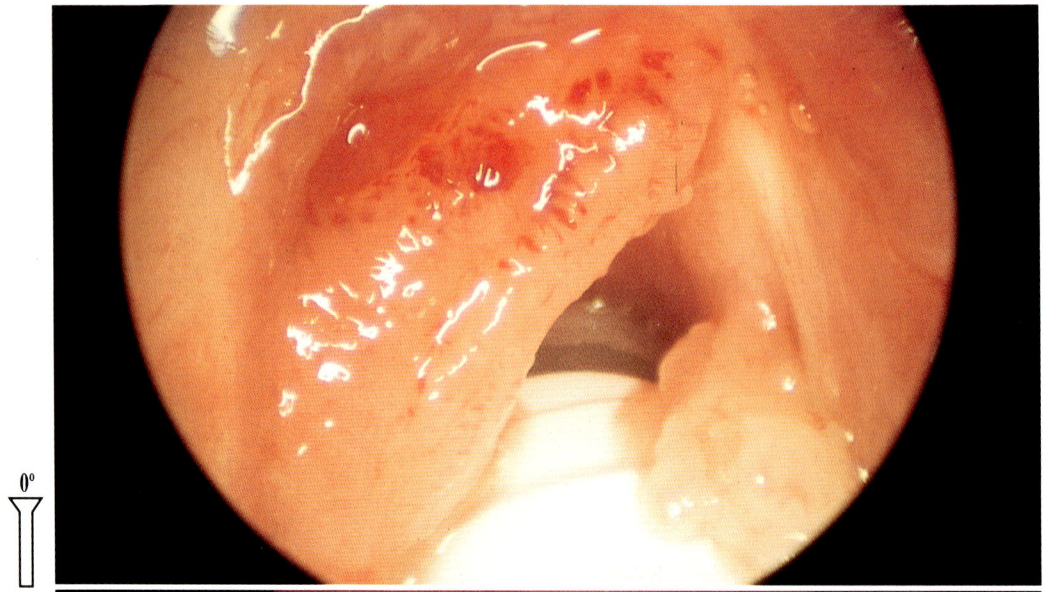
0°

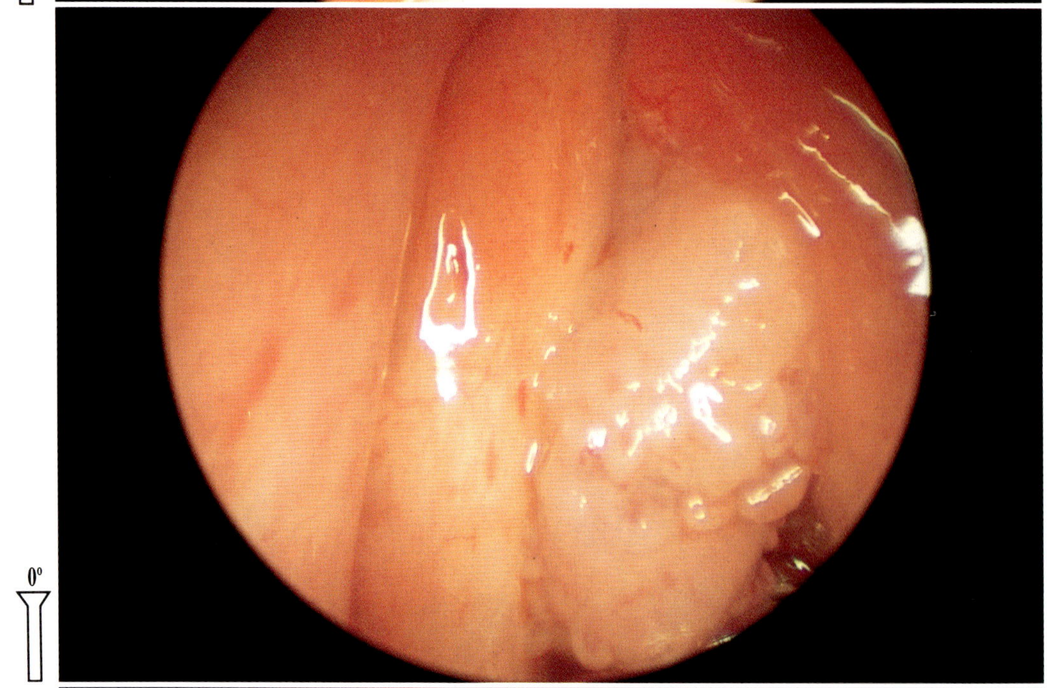
0°

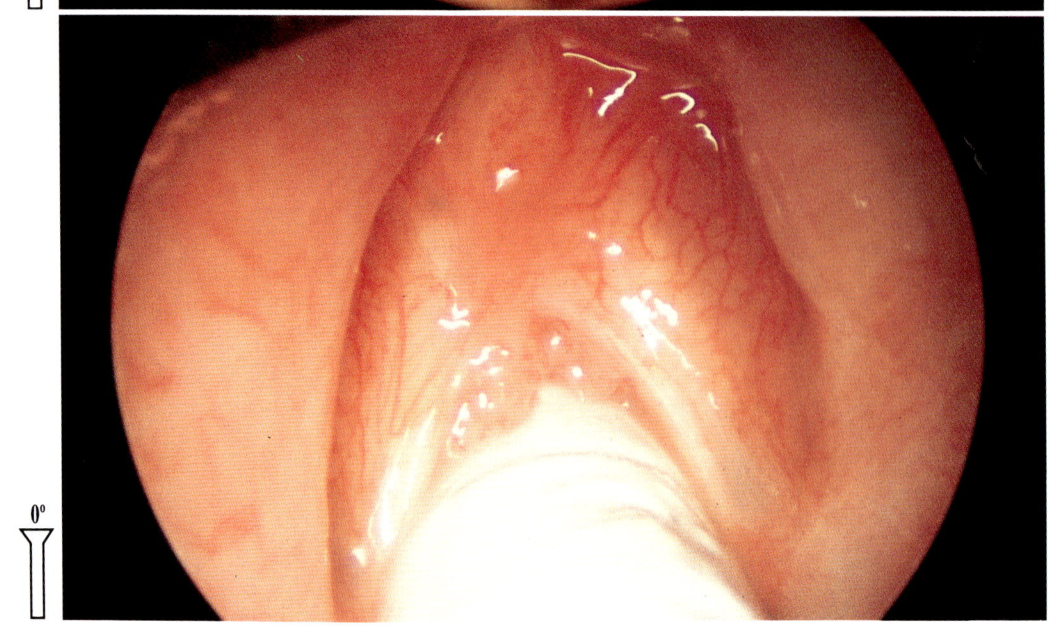
0°

FIG. 48. This 3-year-old boy has juvenile papillomatosis. Papillomas can be seen on the superior surface of the left vocal cord and on its middle and posterior thirds of the right vocal cord.

FIG. 49. This 10-year-old boy has juvenile papillomatosis. The lesion is pedunculated at the middle third of the superior surface of the left vocal cord. The patient has already had several operations.

FIG. 50. This 4-year-old girl has juvenile papillomatosis. There is an anterior commissure synechia with papillomatosis subglottic recidivation.

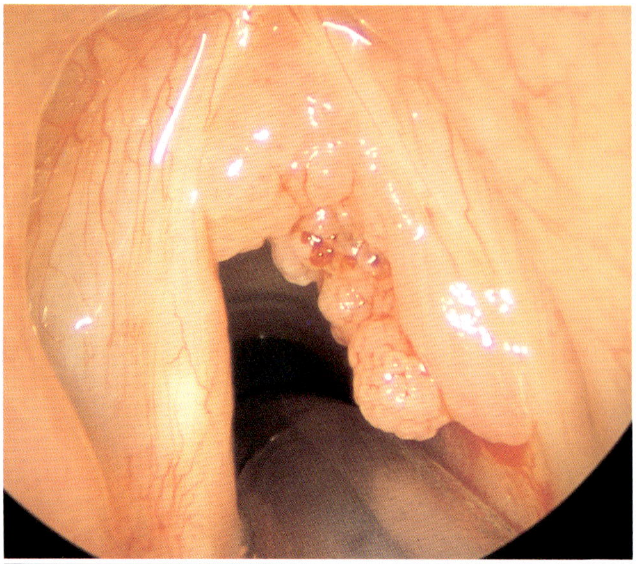

0°

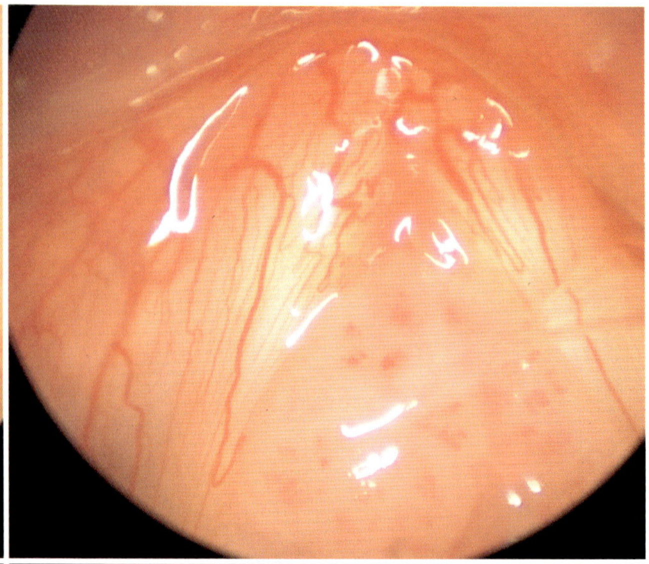

0°

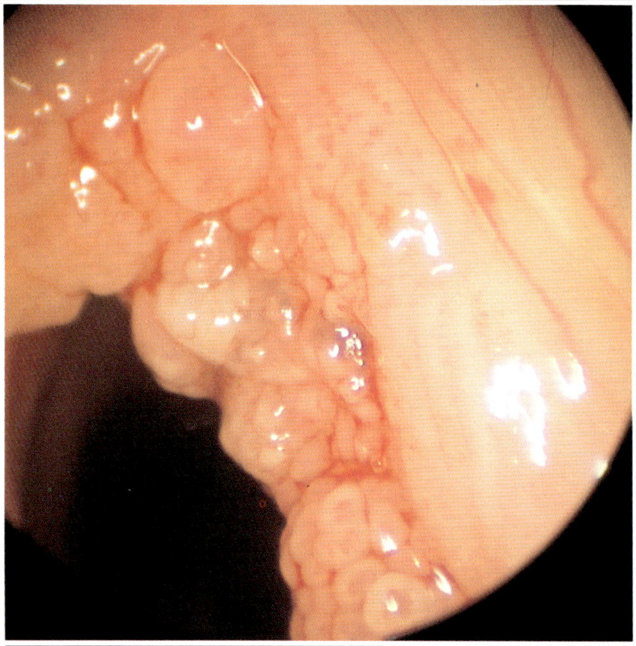

30°

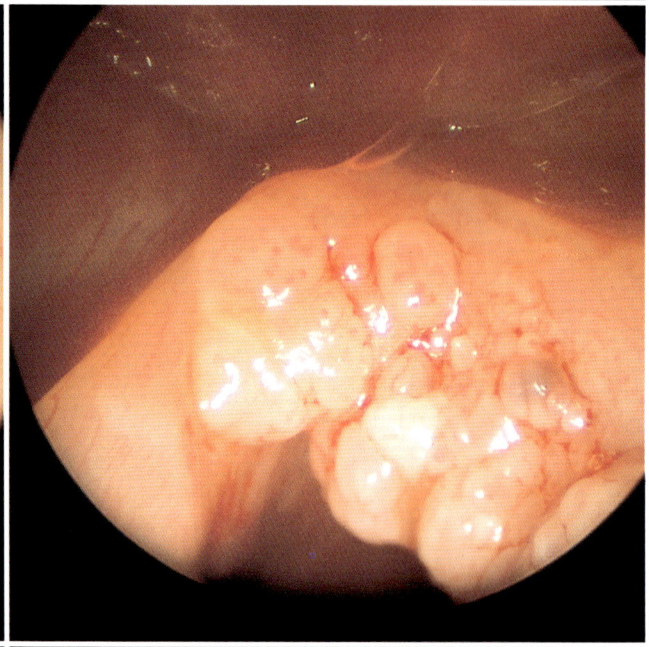

70°

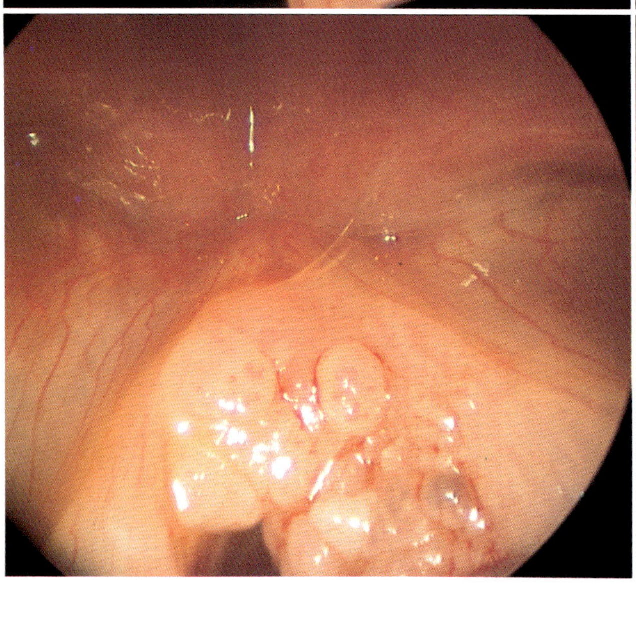

70°

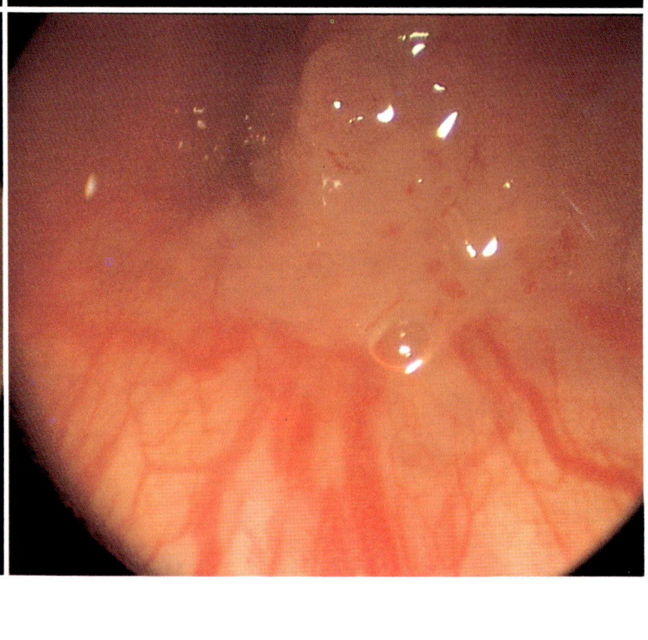

120°

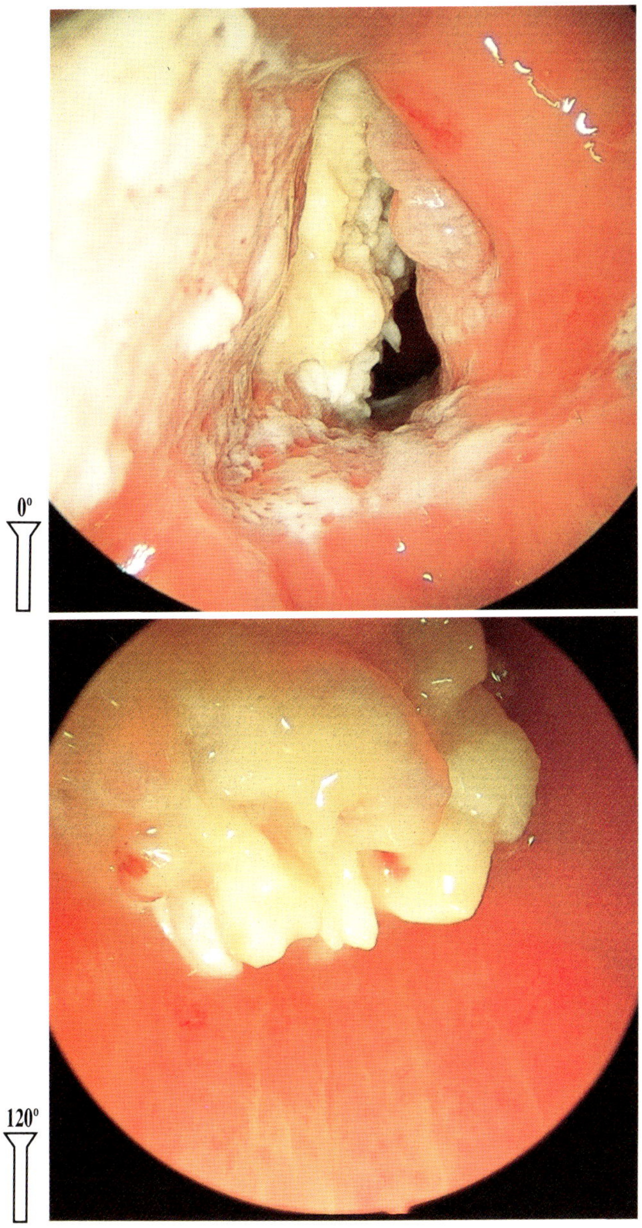

FIG. 52. This large keratotic papilloma occurs in a 45-year-old council officer with a long smoking history. Associated inflammation of the subglottic mucosa is observed with the 120° telescope. There are also signs of a concurrent mycotic infection.

FIG. 51. This 26-year-old man has papilloma occupying the right vocal cord and extending to the subglottis. The lesion goes into the anterior commissure and passes to the anterior part of the left vocal cord. With the 70° and 120° endoscopes, the height of the papilloma and its inferior limit can be seen. The vascular network of the subglottis is abnormally congested.

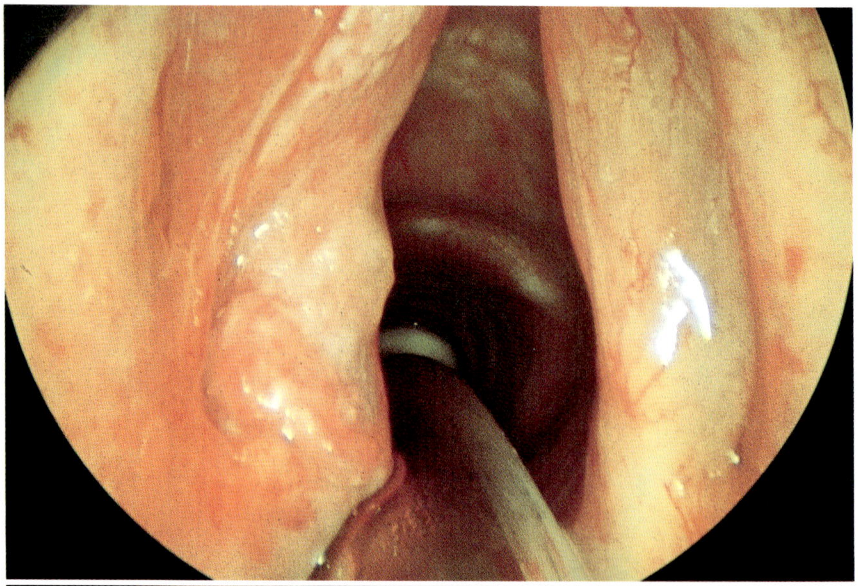

0°

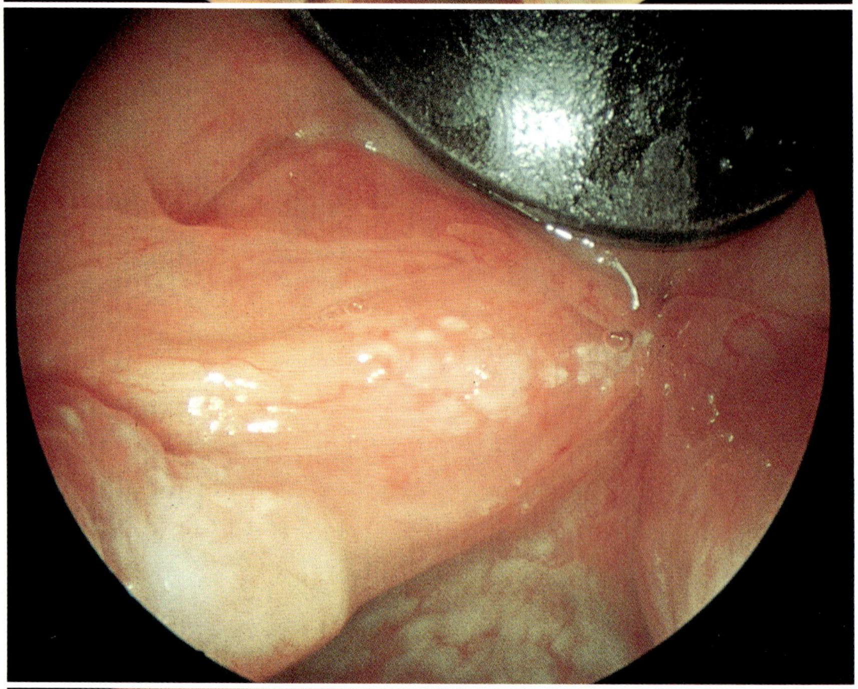

70°

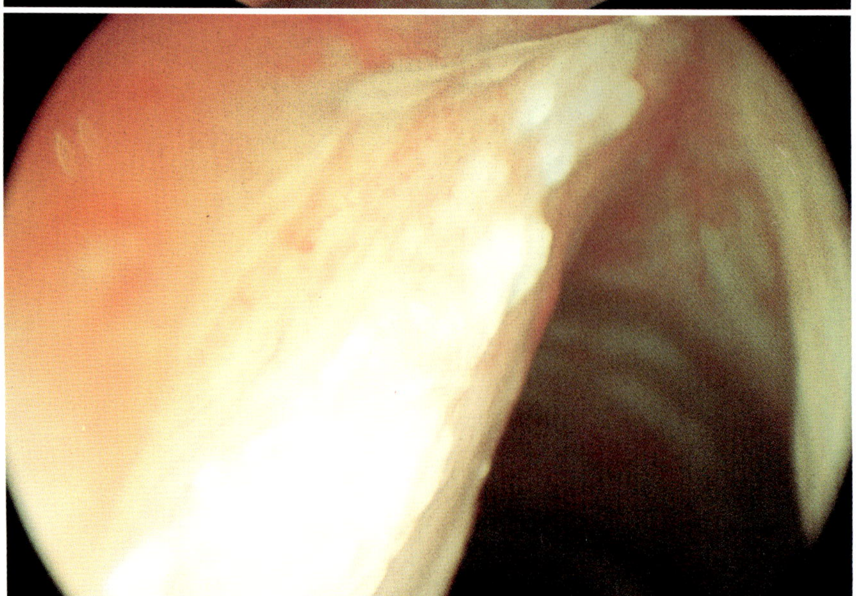

30°

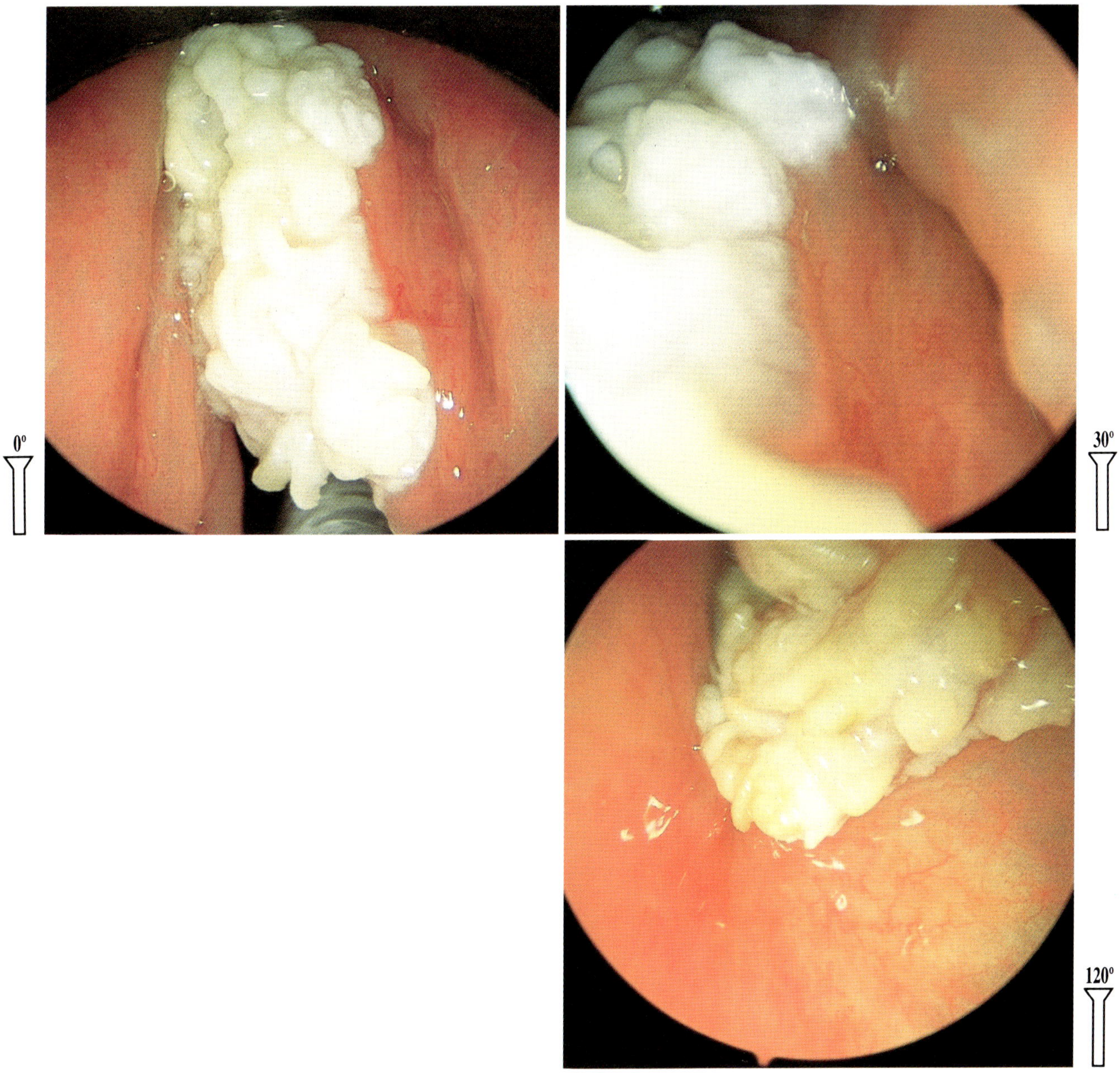

FIG. 54. This keratotic papilloma occurs in a 35-year-old farmer with smoking habits. REMS evaluation contributes to improved assessment of the limits of the lesion and its characteristics. There are signs of intense inflammation at the mucosa of the Ventricle of Morgagni and the subglottis.

FIG. 53. This 61-year-old male has a keratotic papilloma of the left vocal cord. Previous biopsies have revealed chronic inflammation and moderate dysplasia. However, contact endoscopy allows *in vivo* and *in situ* identification of koilocytes. Histological exam confirmed the diagnosis of papilloma.

0°

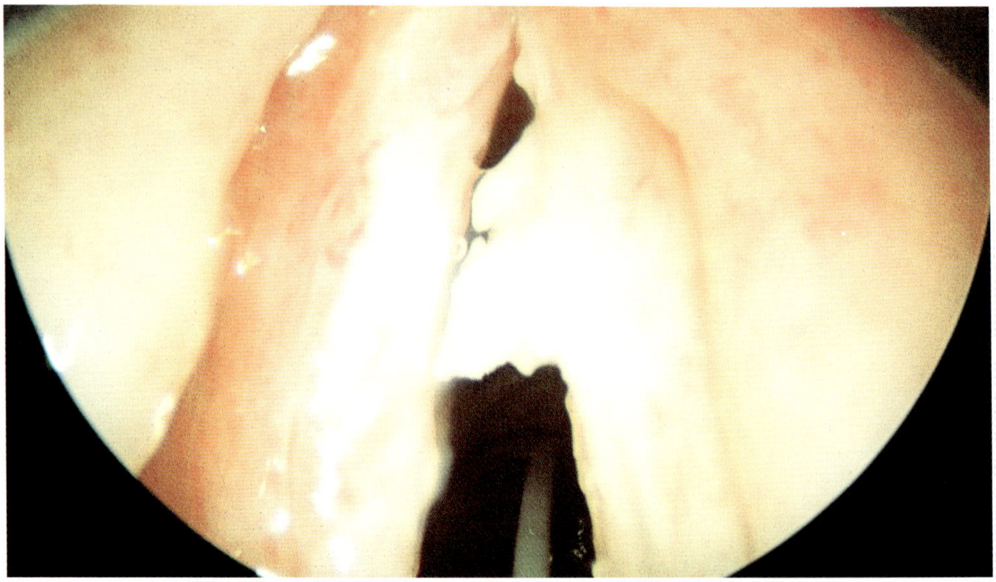

70°

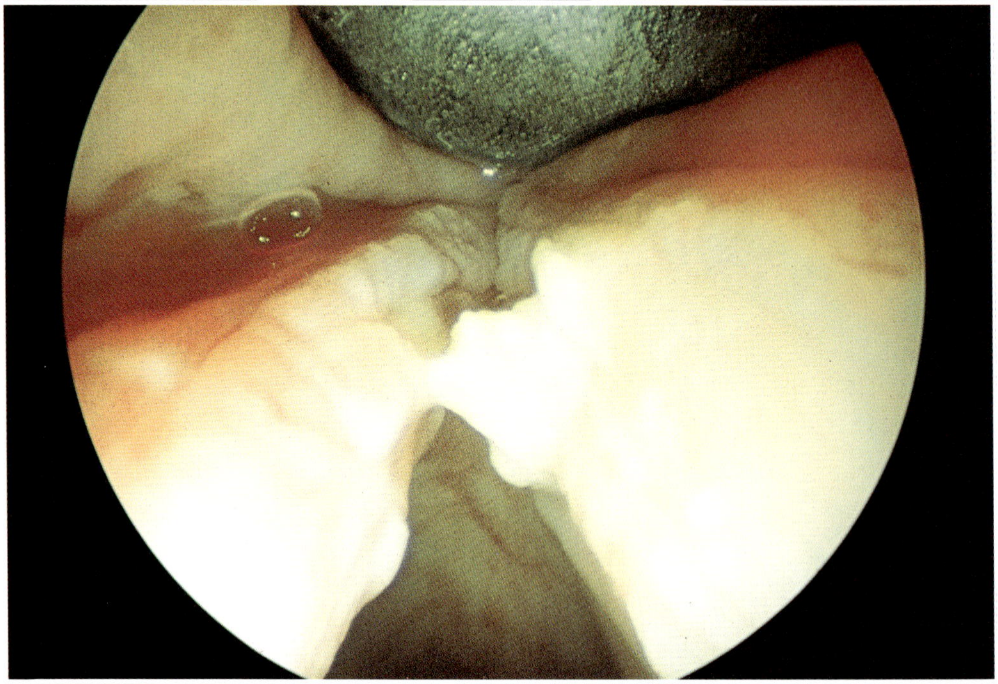

120°

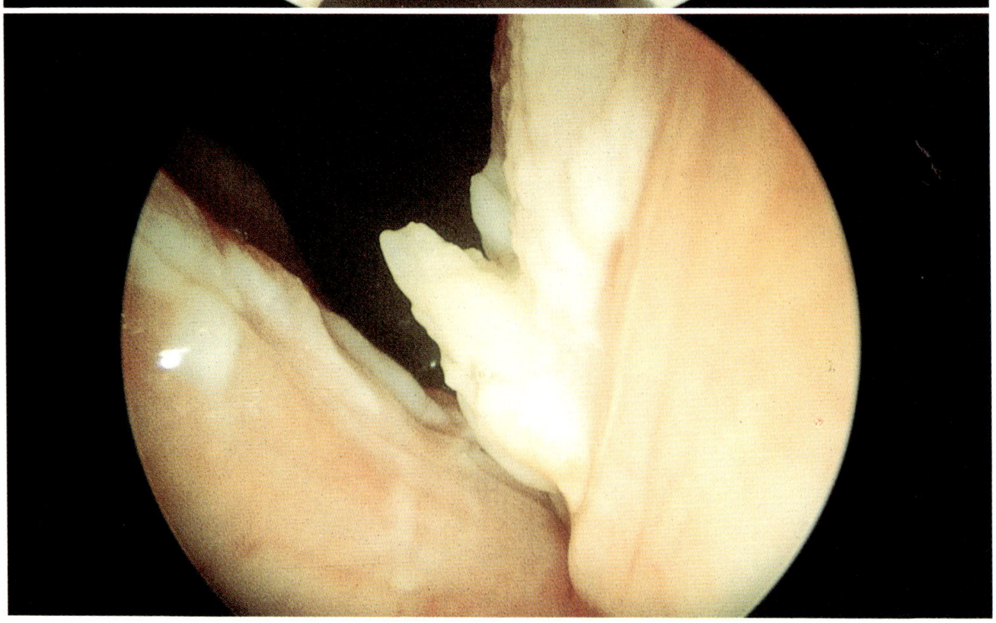

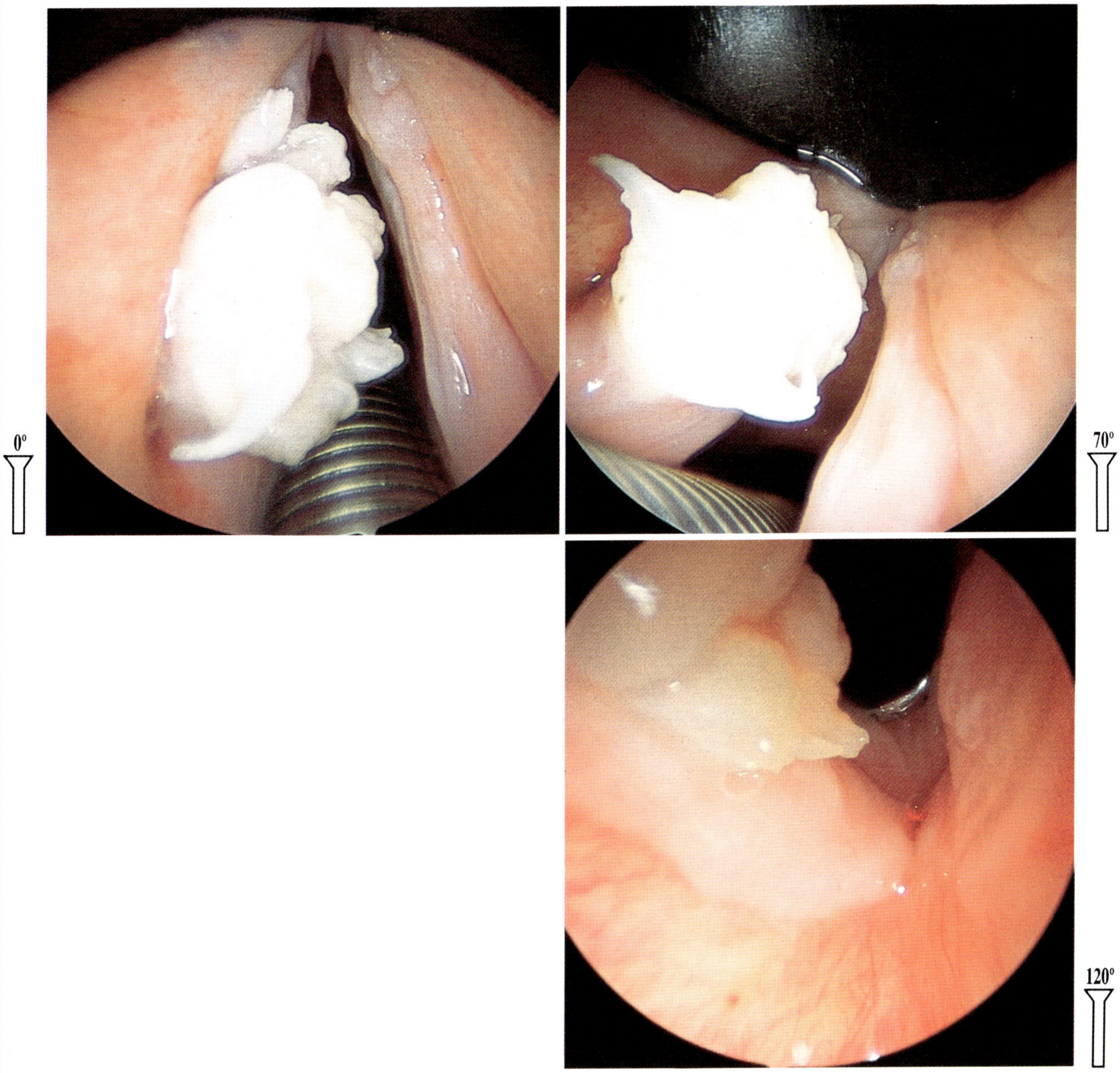

FIG. 56. Left glottic keratotic papilloma observed in a 55-year-old judge. Besides the diagnostic assessment, telescopes allow precise operative control.

←

FIG. 55. This 63-year-old man has keratotic papilloma on both vocal cords. Edema and keratosis are diffuse at the superior and inferior surface of both vocal cords.

REMS also contributes to understanding the evolution of Reinke's edema and its development stage. In some cases, the vasculature of the mucosa is one of the main features; in other cases, queratosis will not allow the observation of the blood vessels. In one case, we were able to diagnose an infiltrating tumor below Reinke's edema that extended into the subglottis. This would not have been detected at that phase if observation had been limited to the superior surface of the vocal cord.

In chronic laryngitis, the difference between microscopic observation and that allowed by the rigid endoscope is significant, as subtle color alterations, relief changes, areas of keratosis, vascular abnormalities, and edema are more objectively defined. Information about these features can be used to guide microsurgical excisions and biopsies.

Studying video endoscopic images obtained in both vocal cords and at the rest of the endolarynx contributes to the understanding of the dynamic process of the disease of the laryngeal mucosa. REMS images associated with contact endoscopy assessment proved different phases of the disease occurred simultaneously.

Assessment of stenosis is also improved with REMS evaluation. In fact, stenosis must be evaluated not only in a horizontal plane but the disease must be considered tridimensionally at different levels of the larynx. The endoscopic multiperspective view in conjunction with CT and MRI provides a better assessment of stenosis.

The surgical technique should be assisted step by step through the endoscopes, choosing the optics according to the stenosed area. In one child, using rigid endoscopes, three separate lesions compromising the airway were identified: a synechia of the posterior commissure, a thin subglottic ring, and a granuloma above the tracheotomy cannula. Of these three, only the first lesion could be observed with the microscope. This patient is presently decanulated.

Rotation of the endoscopes allows a detailed observation in cases of stenosis of the posterior glottis and the height of the arytenoid, which is important in the assessment of granulomas. CO_2 laser arytenoidectomy and posterior cordotomy also benefit with the use of the endoscope.

Laryngeal papillomatosis and papillomas also benefit with the REMS evaluation. The ability to explore the ventricle, the anterior commissure, and the inferior surface of the vocal cord reduces the possibility of residual lesions.

As surgery progresses, the control of the lesion and of its anatomic relationships are clearly evaluated with different optics.

The magnifications and different angles of the endoscopes allow the surgeon to establish a more precise limit of the diseased and the normal mucosa.

If the introduction of the CO_2 laser has improved papillomatosis surgery, the use of endoscopes will also contribute positively to the results.

PREMALIGNANT PATHOLOGY (FIGS. 57–66)

Office endoscopic techniques allow the observation of premalignant pathology at the superior surface of the vocal cord. Microlaryngoscopy makes it possible to observe lesions in better conditions and to perform a biopsy or a microsurgical excision. In benign pathology, REMS allows an overall analysis not only of the lesion that motivated the surgical procedure, but also a very detailed observation of the entire vocal cord.

Frequently, it is noticed that the existence of more than one lesion in areas of the vocal cord is difficult or even impossible to visualize with conventional techniques. Beyond the main lesions, subtle abnormalities at the surface indicate different stages of pathology. The detailed observation with the endoscopes reinforces the physiopathologic notion of a disease that has conceptual repercussions influencing the

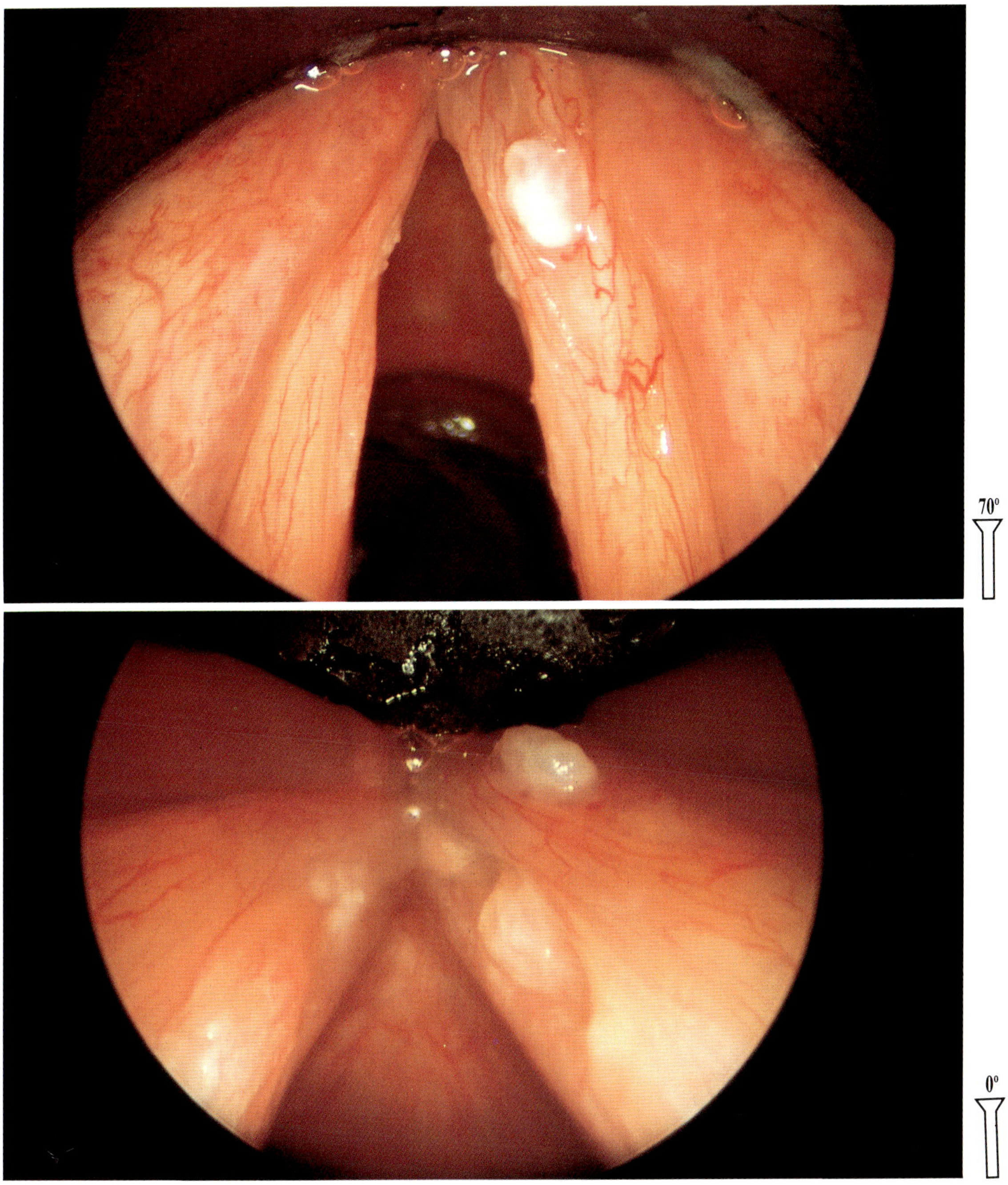

FIG. 57. This 62-year-old man is a cigarette smoker and merchant. There is leukoplakia with well defined limits at the superior surface of the right vocal cord. The relief of the leukoplakia is better evaluated with the 70° endoscope. There are significant differences in the vasculature of the superior surface of both vocal cords. With the 70° endoscope, other keratotic lesions situated at the free border of the vocal cords can be seen clearly.

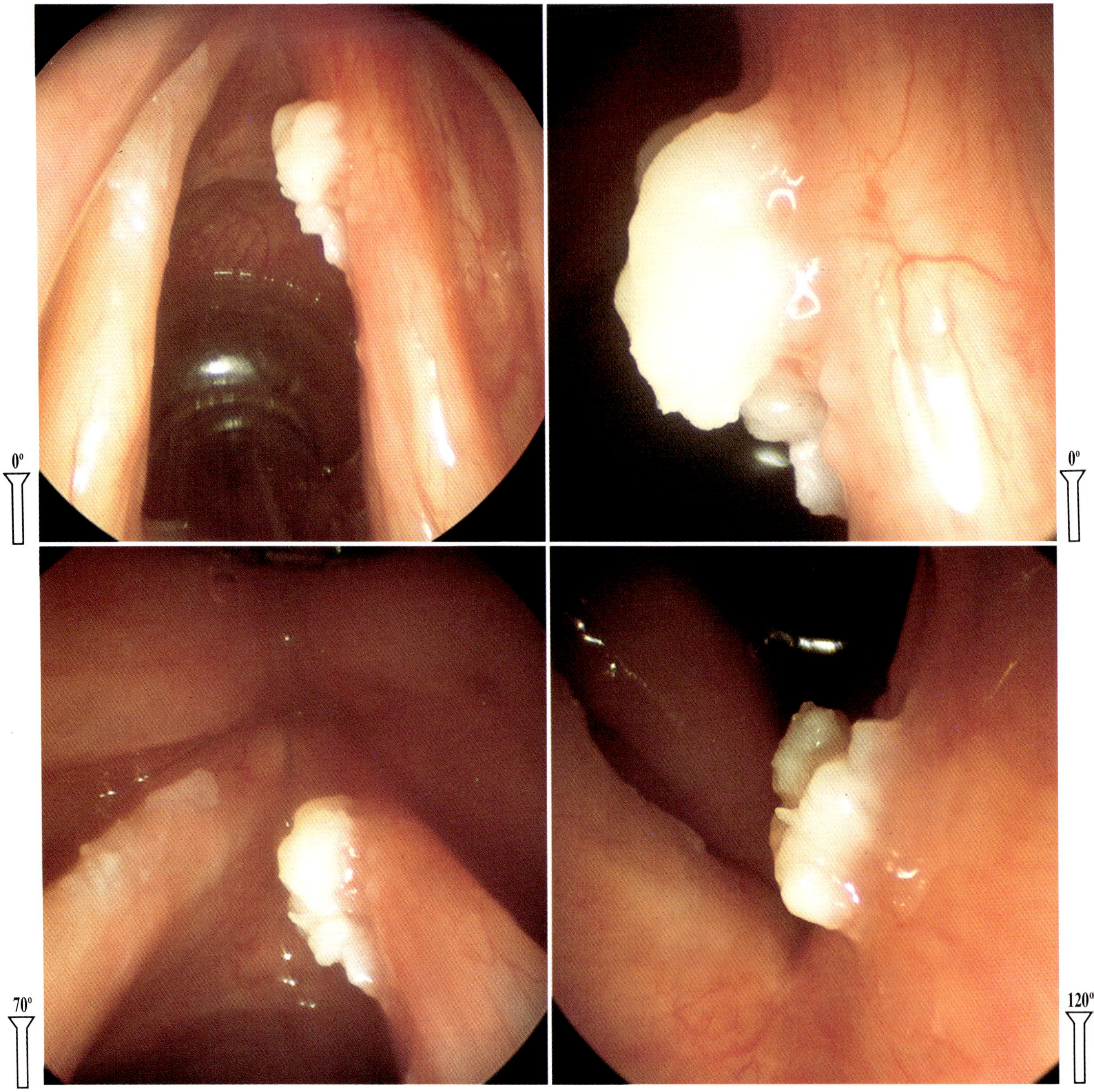

FIG. 58. This 66-year-old man is a cigarette smoker and a farmer. There is leukoplakia at the free border of the right vocal cord. The height of the lesion and its inferior surface are assessed with 70° and 120° endoscopes. At the superior surface there are alterations of the blood vessels surrounding the leukoplakia. At the left vocal cord there is another leukoplakia with distinct characteristics.

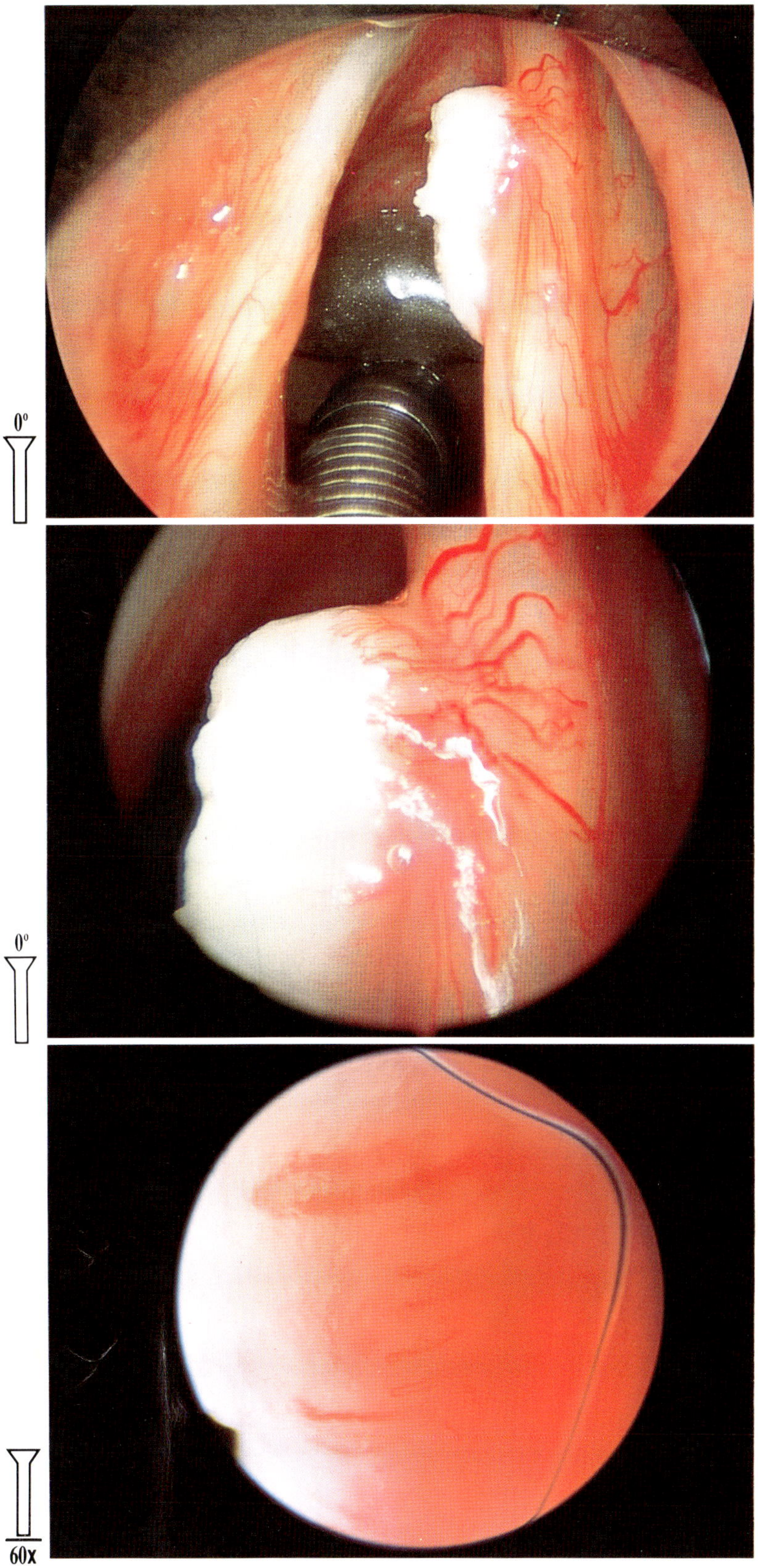

FIG. 59. One year post-op images of the patient described in Fig. 58. There is a recurrence of hyperkeratosis on the right vocal cord. With the high magnifications obtained with these endoscopes, it is possible to demonstrate the vascular arcades at the base of the lesion, typical of papilloma. The lower image was obtained with contact endoscopy.

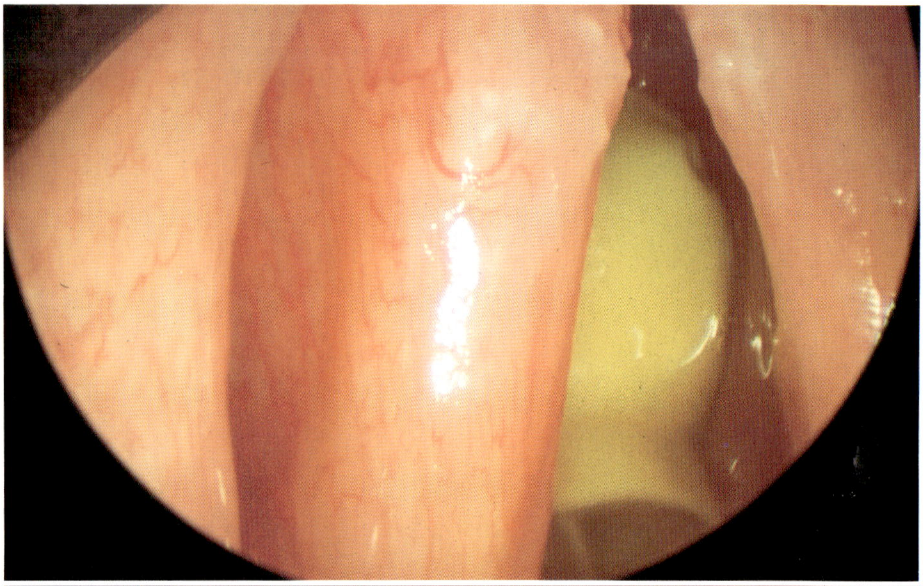

0°

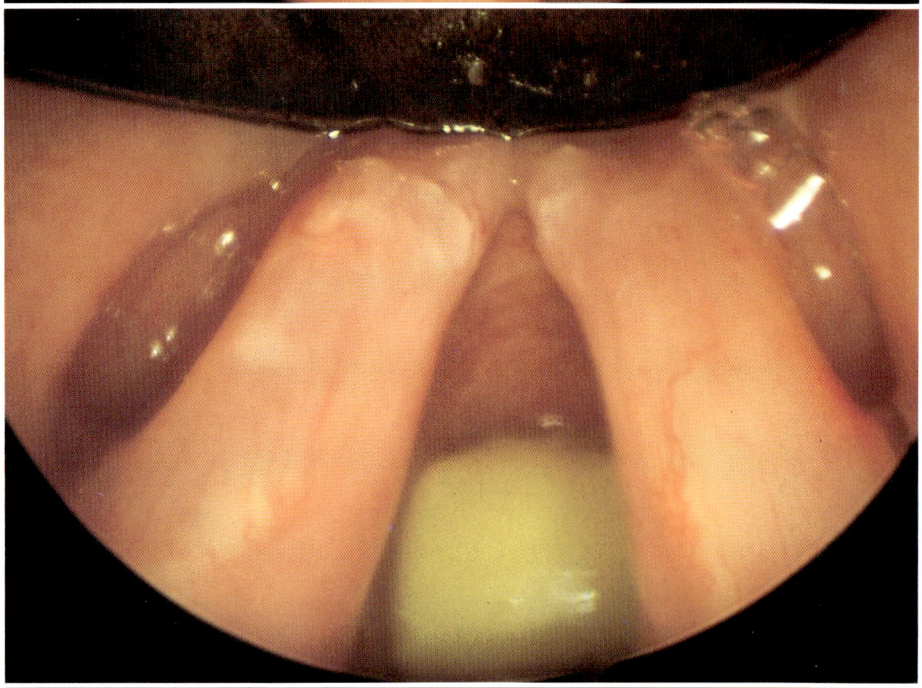

70°

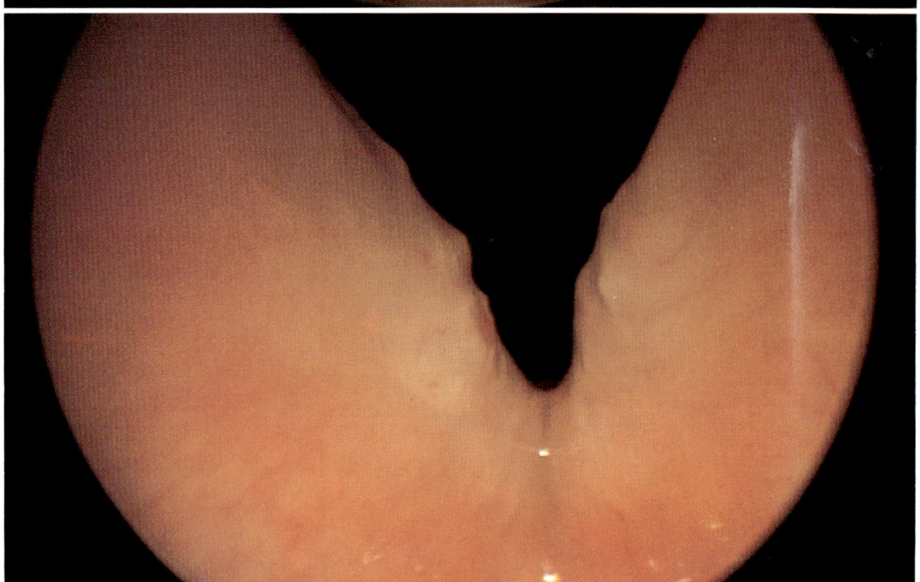

120°

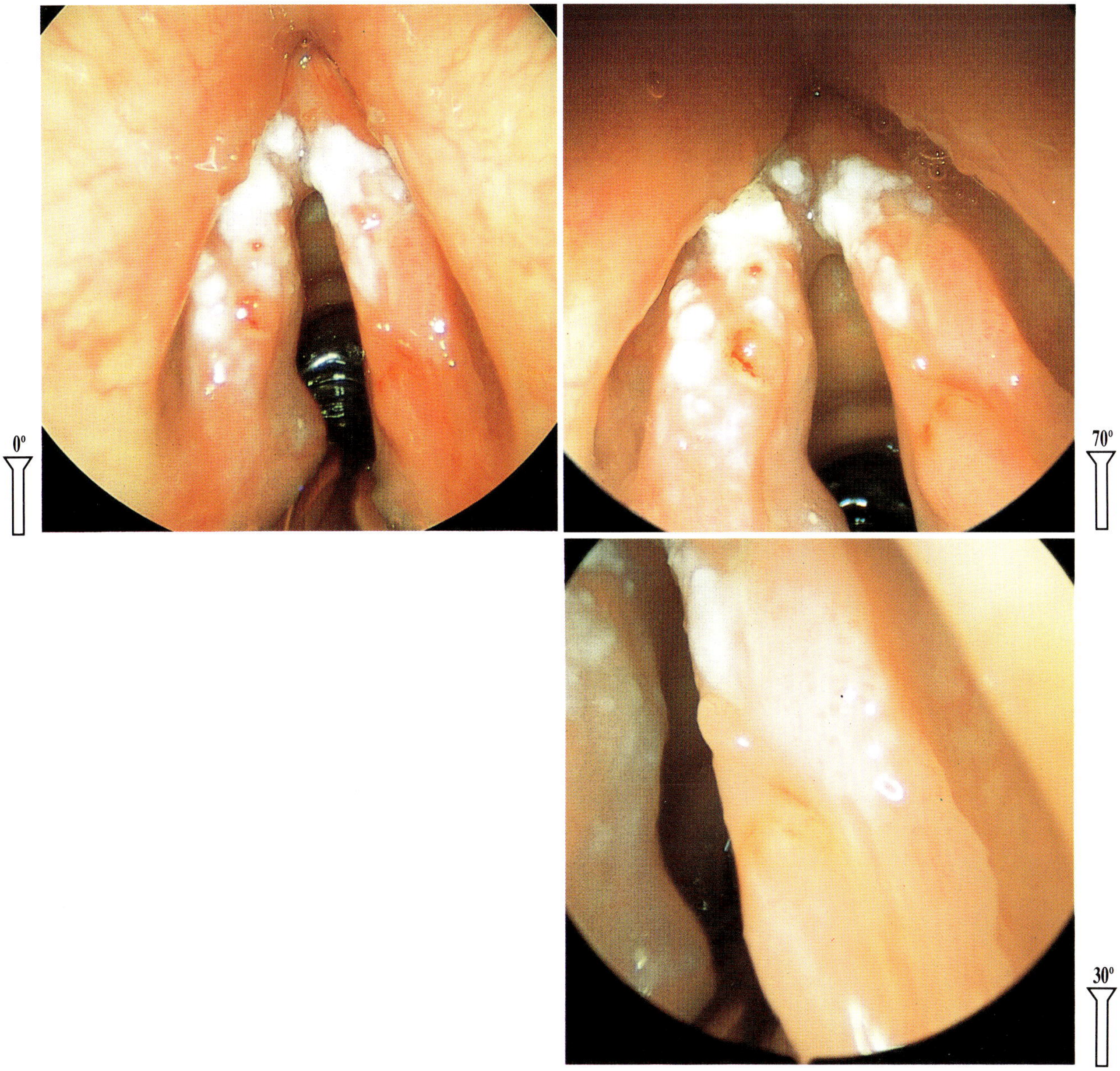

FIG. 61. This is a 57-year-old farmer, with a history of tobacco abuse. On both vocal cords there are scattered areas of keratosis, edema, and vascular changes associated with papilloma.

FIG. 60. This 35-year-old man is a cigarette smoker and a bricklayer. He has lesions of leukoplakia on both vocal cords. On the left side there are already vascular alterations around the leukoplakia. The relief of the leukoplakia is more evident using the 70° telescope. Different degrees of keratosis are observed along the surface of the vocal cords. With the 120° telescopes, it can be seen that the keratosis extends to the inferior surface of the vocal cords.

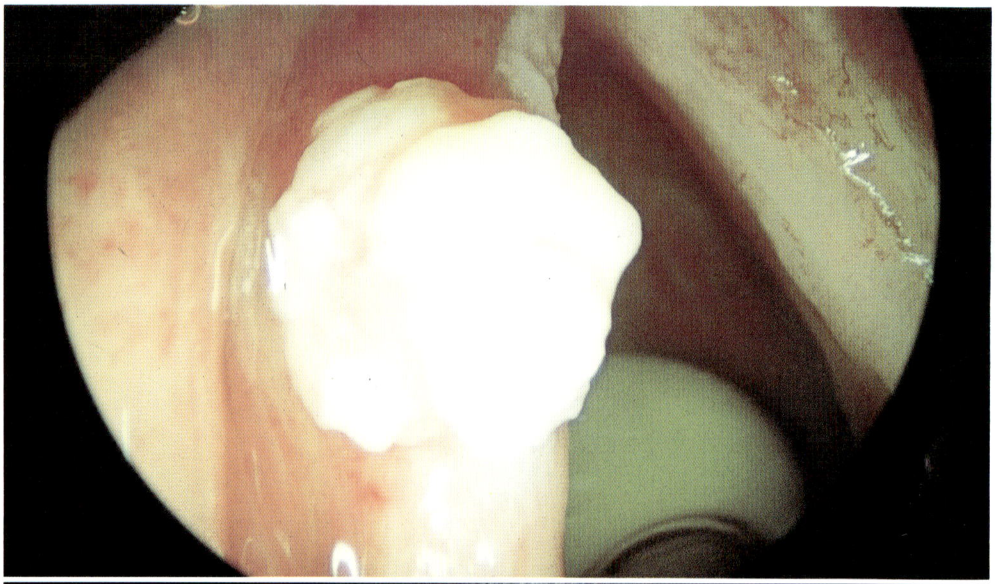

0°

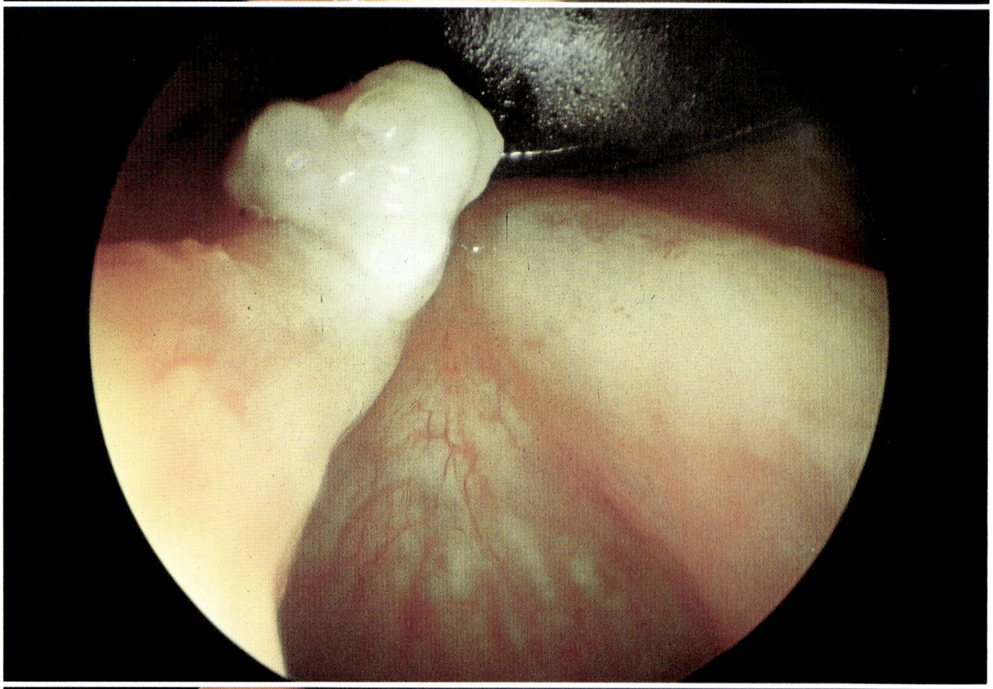

70°

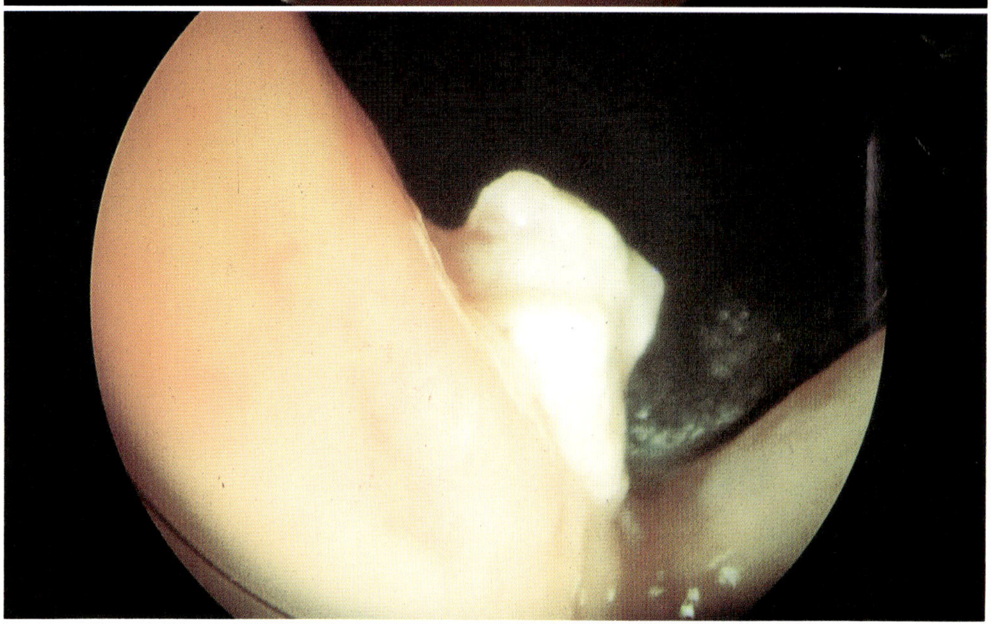

120°

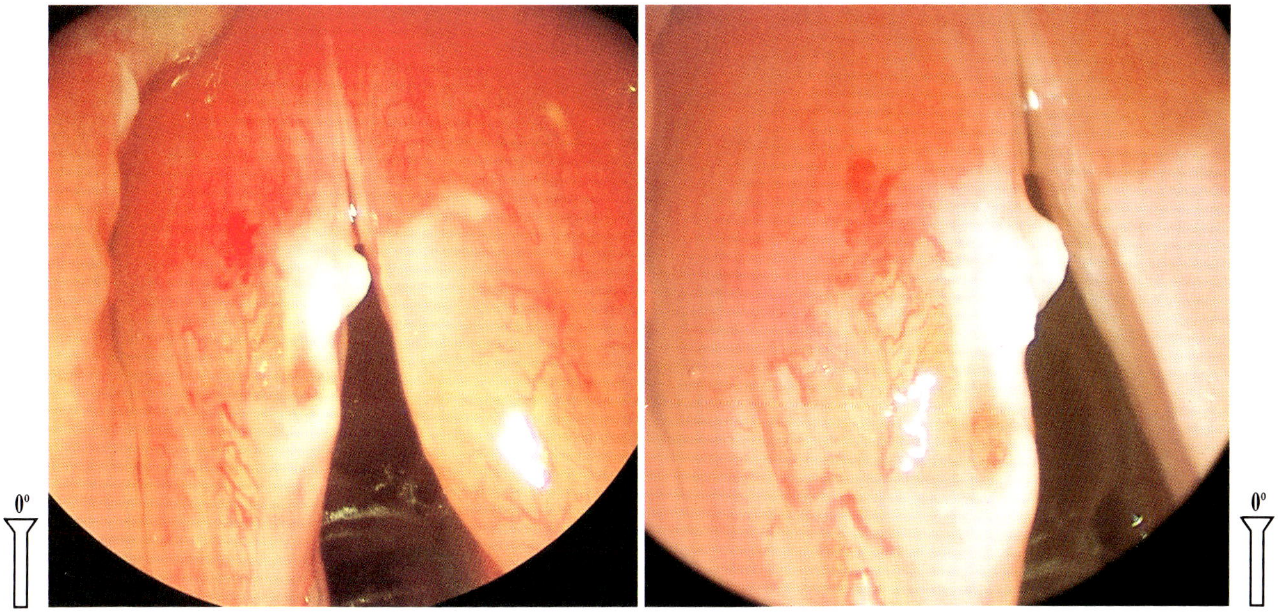

FIG. 63. This is a 45-year-old railway worker with a history of tobacco abuse. Areas of keratosis, edema, and severe vascular changes are present on both vocal cords. Endoscopes allow good visualization of mucosal characteristics and support the concept of laryngeal disease with different phases occuring simultaneously in the same patient.

FIG. 62. This 48-year-old man is a cigarette smoker and a bricklayer. There is a keratotic lesion implanted at the middle third of the free border and superior surface of the vocal cord. Keratosis extends to the anterior commissure. On the right vocal cord keratinization is less pronounced.

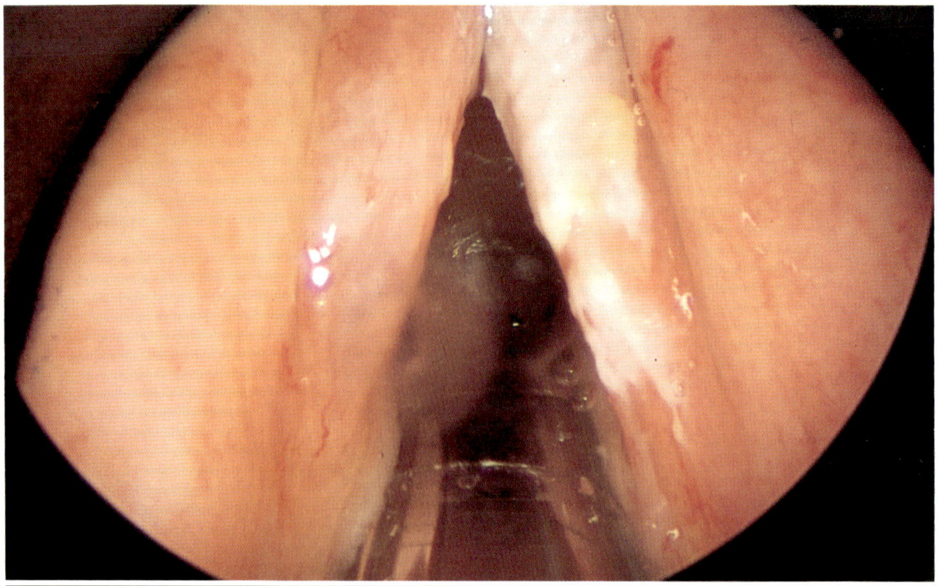

0°

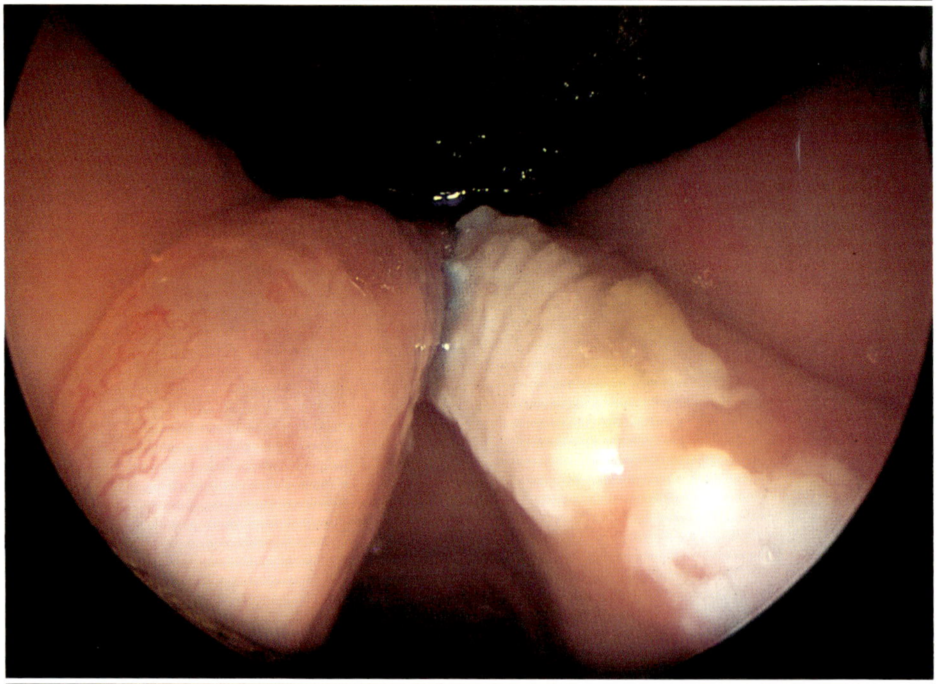

70°

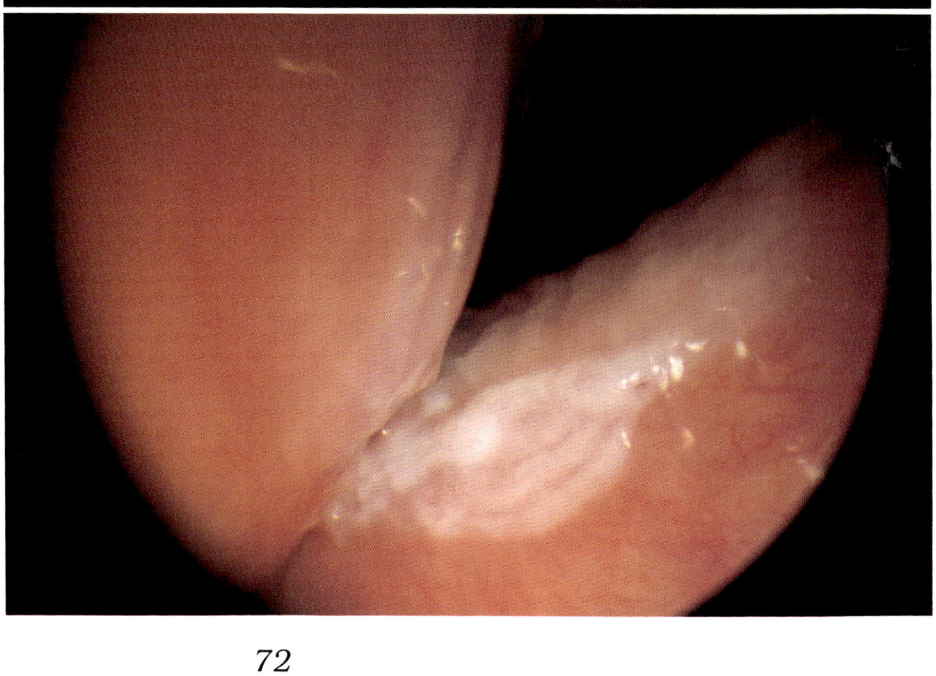

120°

0°

70°

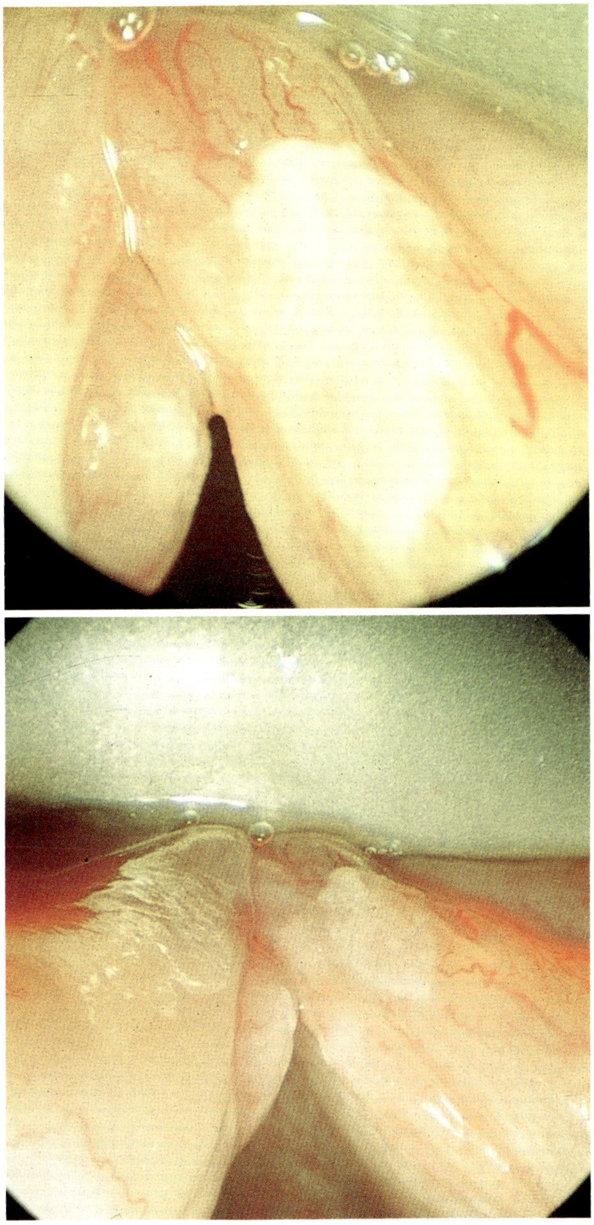

FIG. 65. This 51-year-old football referee with a history of smoking exhibits leukoplakia localized to the anterior right vocal cord. This is associated with polyps in early development at the free borders of both vocal cords. Diffuse edema and vascular changes are also noted.

FIG. 64. This 69-year-old man is a cigarette smoker. There is an extensive keratotic lesion covering the superior and inferior surface of the right vocal cord. Use of the 70° and 120° endoscopes accentuates the relief of the leukoplakia and contributes to a more complete topographic assessment. The left vocal cord shows inflammatory signs of chronic inflammation with less keratosis.

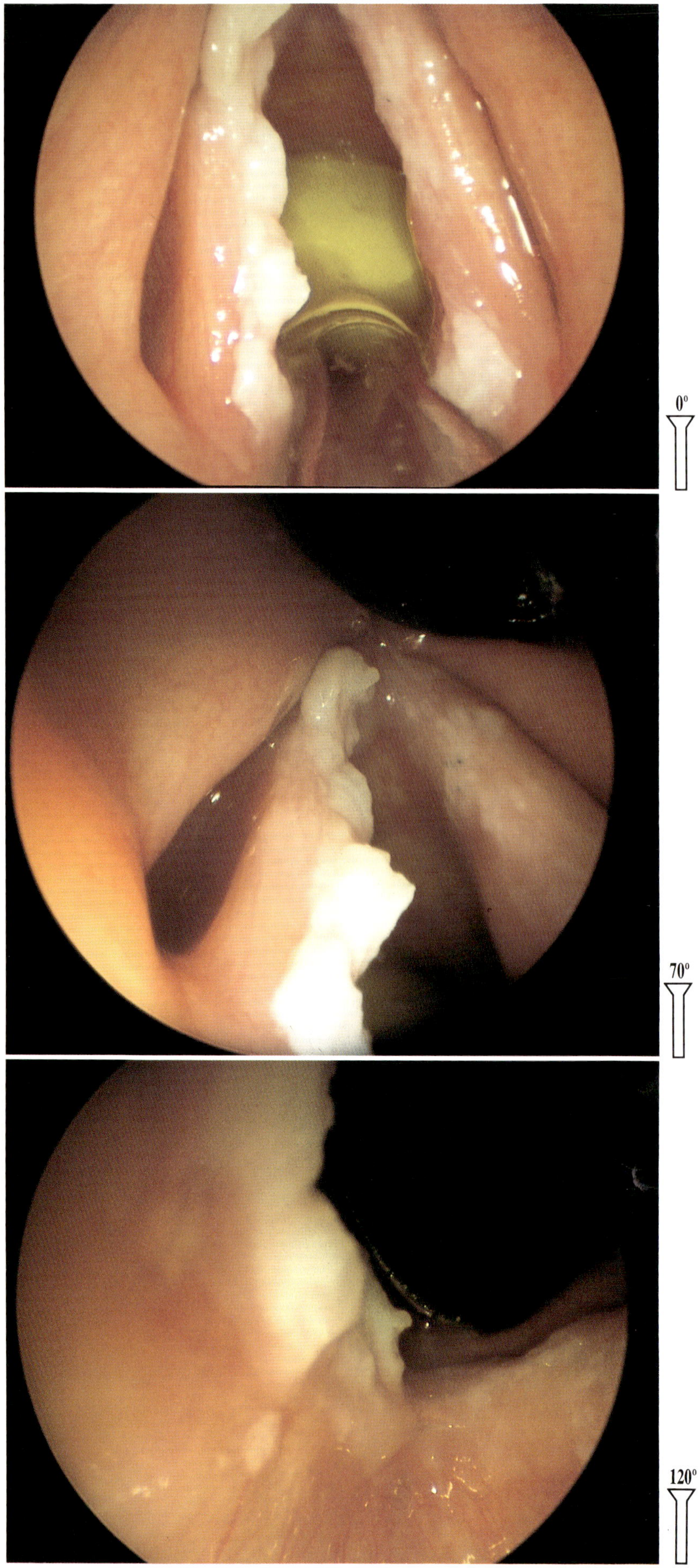

FIG. 66. This 64-year-old man is a cigarette smoker. Extensive keratotic lesions occupy the left vocal cord and extend to its inferior surface. On the right side, keratinization is diffuse but in an earlier phase of development.

therapeutic approach and the pathological control. Besides the inventory of the distinct lesions, REMS offers the possibility of analyzing—dimensions, limits, transition areas to normal mucosa, edemas, surface characteristics, and definition of the vascular pattern. Relief perception is improved with the 30°, 70°, and 120° endoscopes and provides a better definition of the site and the distance that separates lesions from distinct laryngeal landmarks. The 70° and 120° endoscopes allow the surgeon to visualize the leukoplakia when it extends to the free border and to the inferior surface of the vocal cord.

Image processing has important potential applications in this area. Attempts at using computer image processing systems to enhance the analysis of endoscopic images are very promising, allowing the quantification of parameters such as dimensions, contours, and the mapping of the lesions in the endolarynx.

MALIGNANT PATHOLOGY (Figs. 67–79)

If the value of rigid endoscopes has been demonstrated in non-malignant pathology, its importance is even greater in oncology. REMS allows enhanced diagnostic precision in the initial phases of malignant tumors and a precise topographic assessment for the therapeutic approach. Dimensions, shape, boundaries, vascular abnormalities, and evaluation of neighboring regions may be accurately assessed with the 0°, 30°, 70°, and 120° endoscopes.

In a vocal cord tumor classified as a T_1, it is fundamental to evaluate its eventual extension to the inferior surface and to the subglottis. Mobility may not be impaired; CT may not show any abnormality; stroboscopy may already show alterations, but the combined use of the endoscopes allows a more correct evaluation. Endoscopes are critical for the exploration of the potential tumor spreading to regions considered traditionally difficult to assess such as the anterior commissure, and to perform a correct evaluation of regions impossible to observe correctly when using conventional office endoscopic techniques and the microscope—Morgagni ventricle, the inferior surface of the vocal cord, and the subglottis.

The macroscopic characteristics of the tumor—infiltrating, ulcerative, etc.—is another parameter that the endoscopes allow the surgeon to explore. This is particularly evident in the tumors of the laryngeal surface of the epiglottis.

In these tumors, microscopic observation is always limited and can even be impaired by the placement of the laryngoscope. The 70° endoscope (in some cases it is preferable to use 4 mm endoscopes) can provide an excellent view of tumors spreading to the pre-epiglottic space. The same happens with the tumors of the false cord and of the Morgagni ventricle.

The assessment of the majority of these tumors is more precise with CT and in some cases MRI. However, imaging techniques are complementary exams, while endoscopy, even under general anesthesia, is an observation technique.

TNM classification in the larynx shows several limitations, but endoscopy associated with imaging techniques will improve the accuracy of staging.

Performance of different types of (endoscopic/external) partial surgery is also improved with the assistance of video endoscopic per-operative control.

The control of results after partial surgery, radiotherapy, and chemotherapy is much more detailed using the endoscopes.

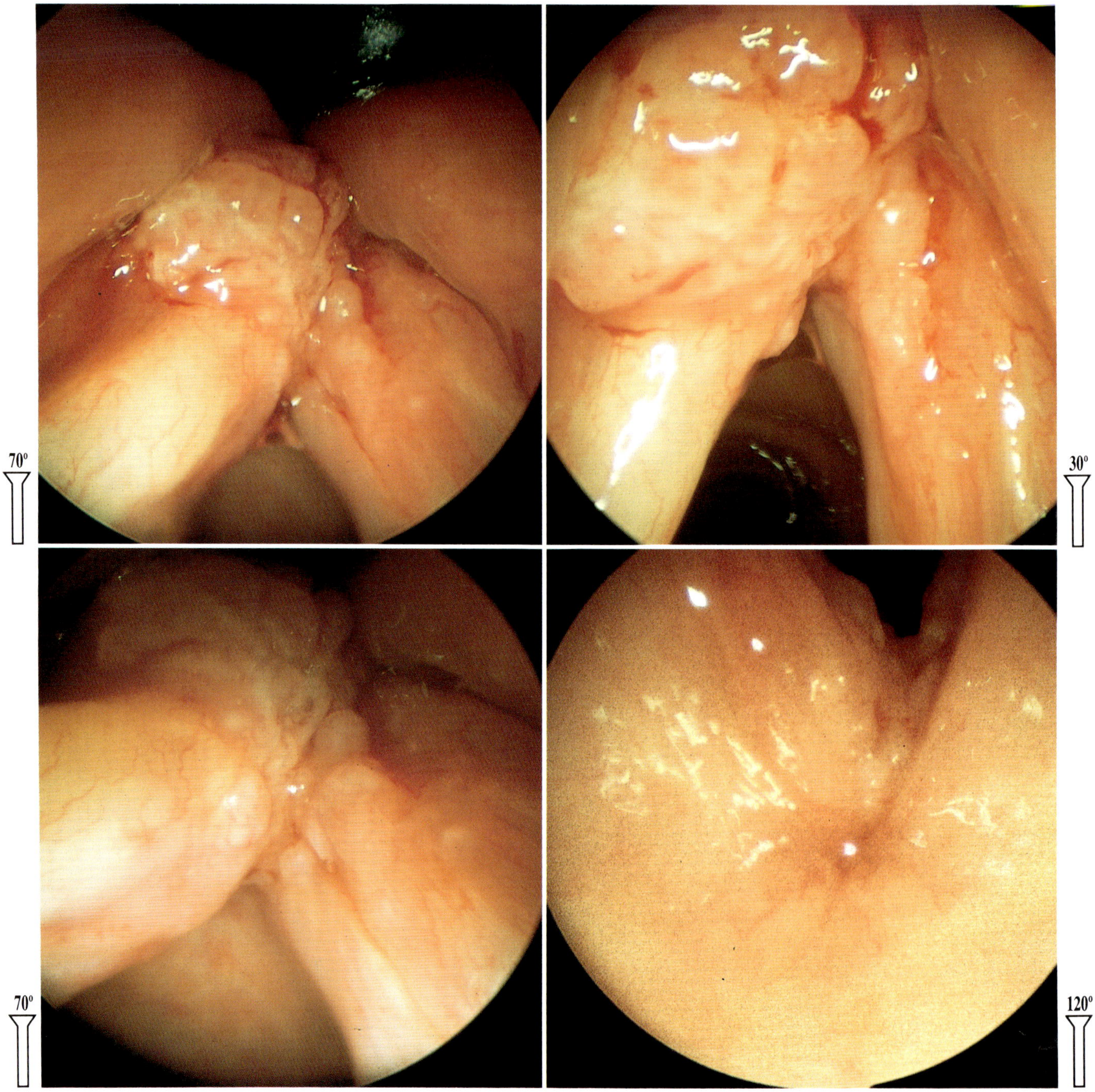

FIG. 67. This 82-year-old man is a cigarette smoker. He has a tumor of the anterior commissure and anterior third of both vocal cords. On the left side, it extends to the anterior part of the Morgagni ventricle, as is evident with the 70° endoscope. The height of the tumor and the inferior extension are assessed with the 70° and 120° endoscopes. The left side of the subglottis is pushed by the tumor.

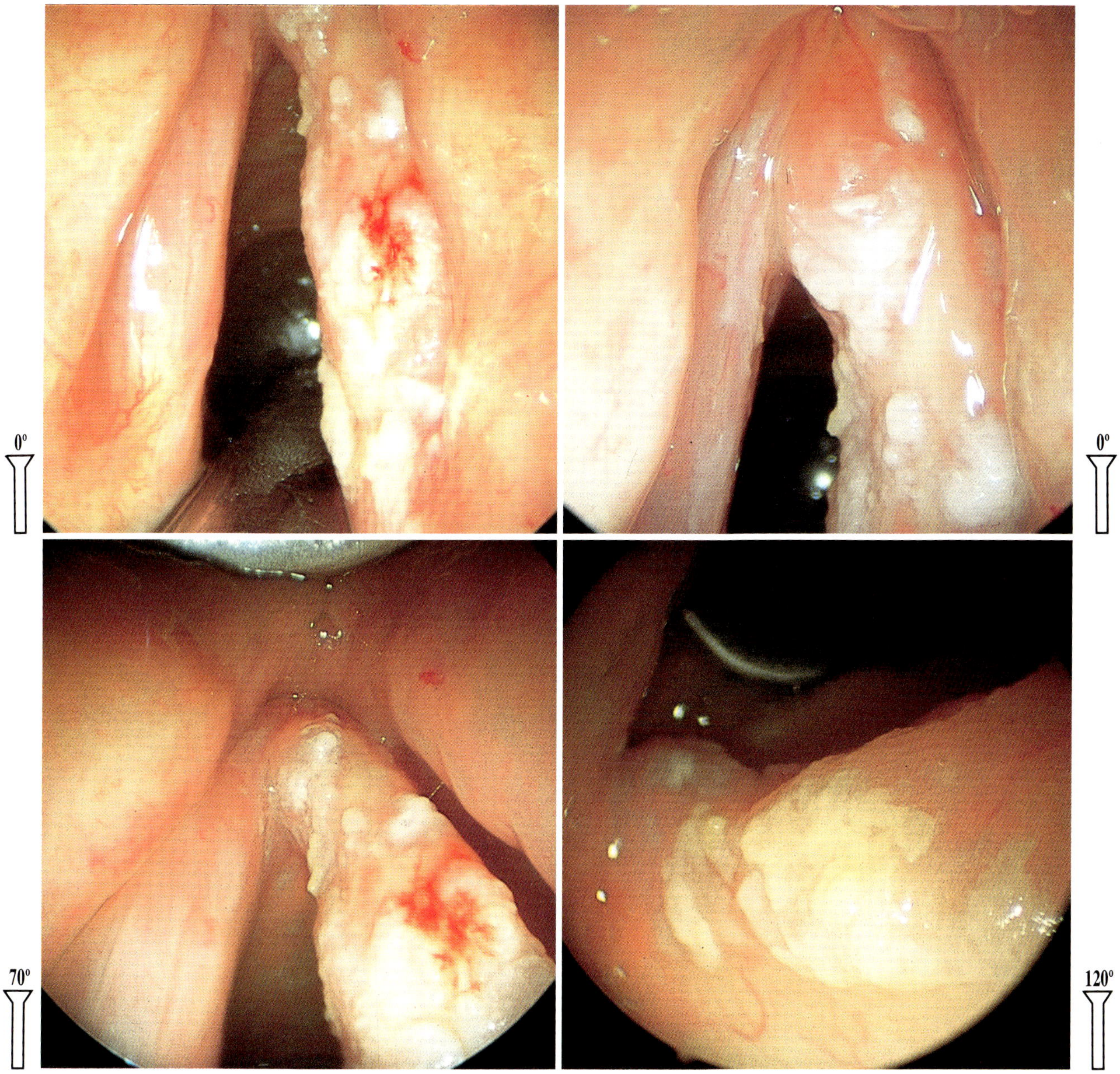

FIG. 68. This 61-year-old patient works in the plastic industry and has a heavy smoking history. There is a malignant tumor along the right vocal cord. Key points in tumor staging, including invasion of the anterior commissure, ventricle, arytenoid and inferior surface of the vocal cord are easily visualized with the telescopes.

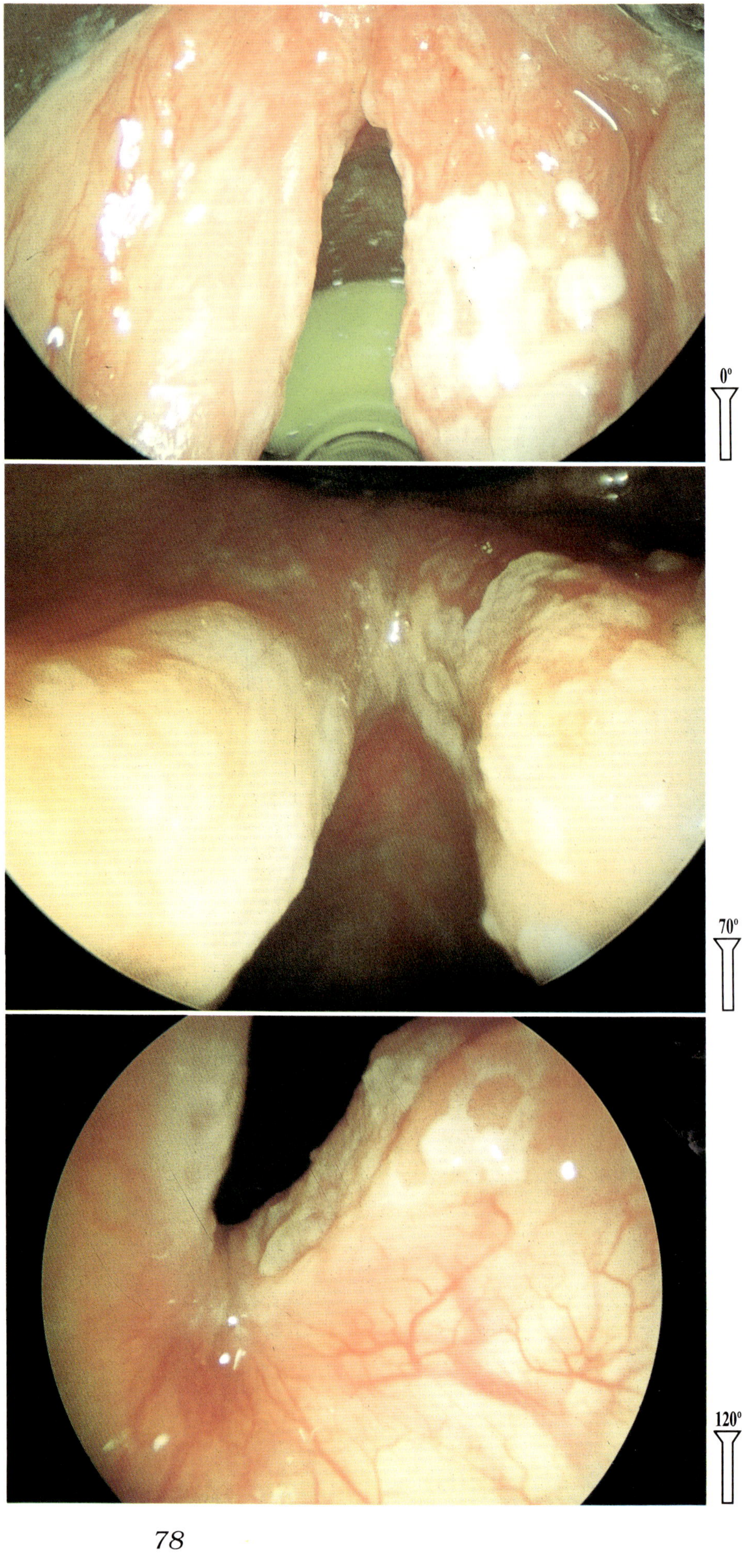

FIG. 69. This 41-year-old man is a cigarette smoker. Carcinoma of both vocal cords can be seen with the 0°, 70°, and 120° telescopes.

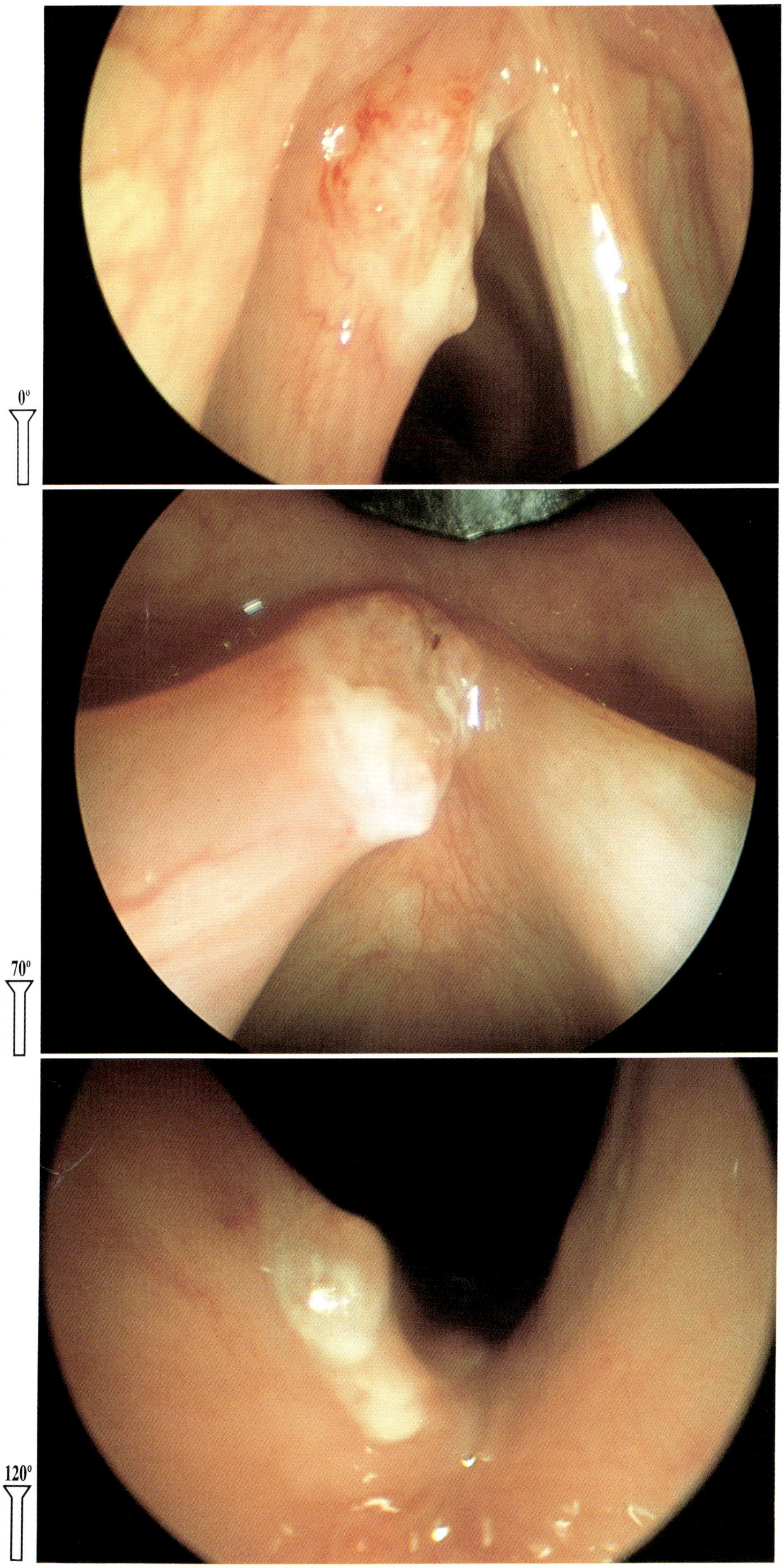

FIG. 70. This 60-year-old salesman is a cigarette smoker. Carcinoma of the anterior third of the left vocal cord is viewed with the 0°, 70°, and 120° telescopes, which allow a multiperspective assessment.

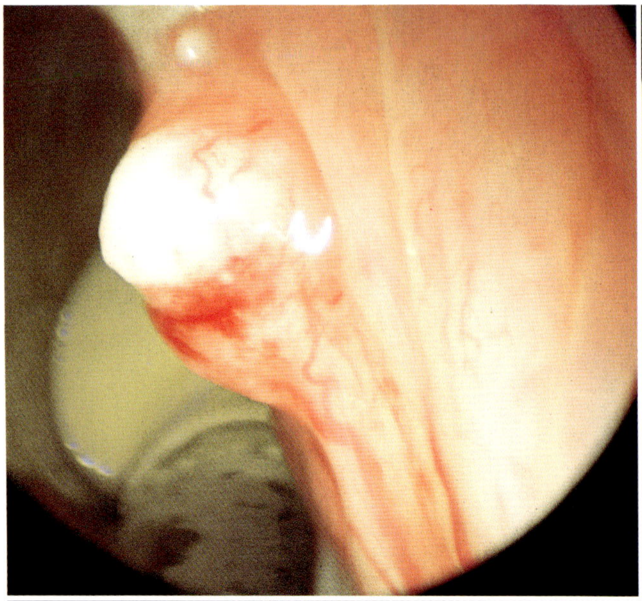

0°

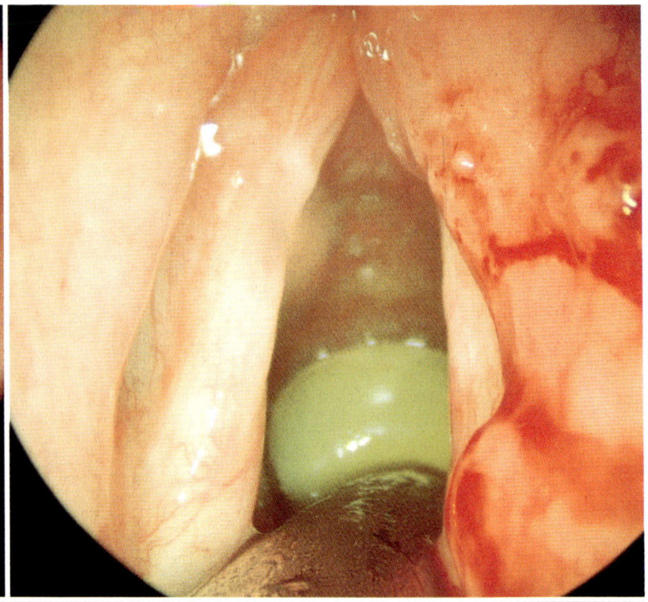

0°

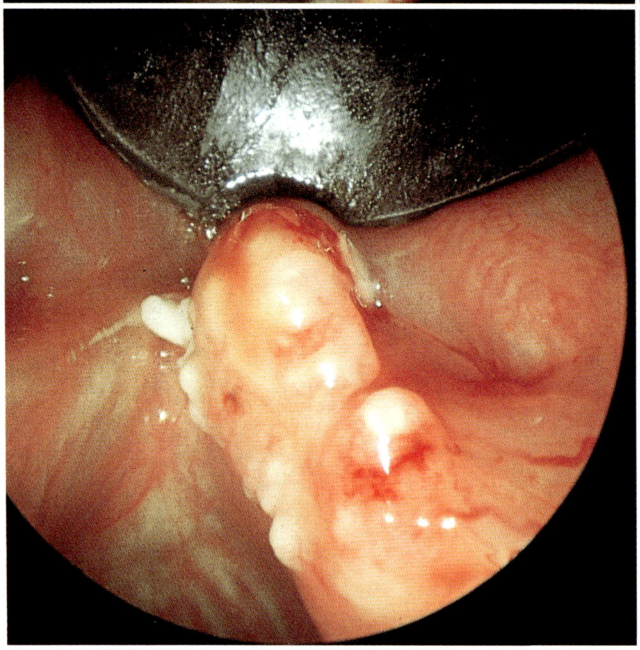

70°

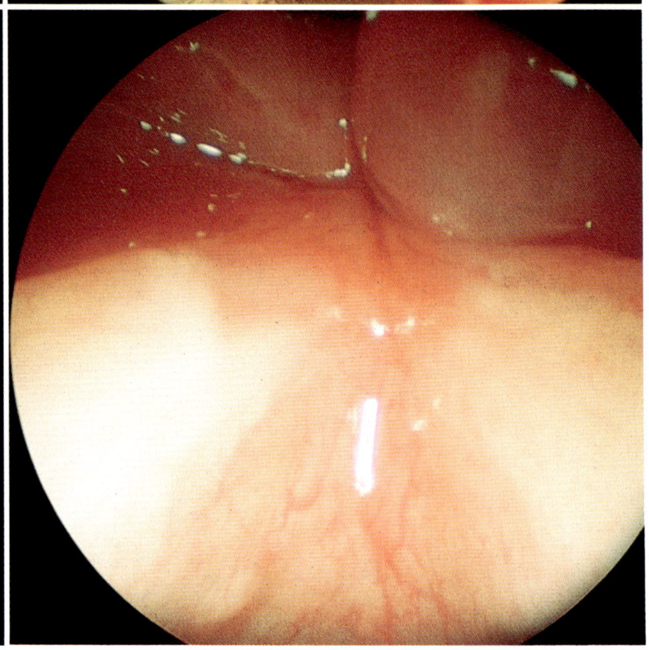

70°

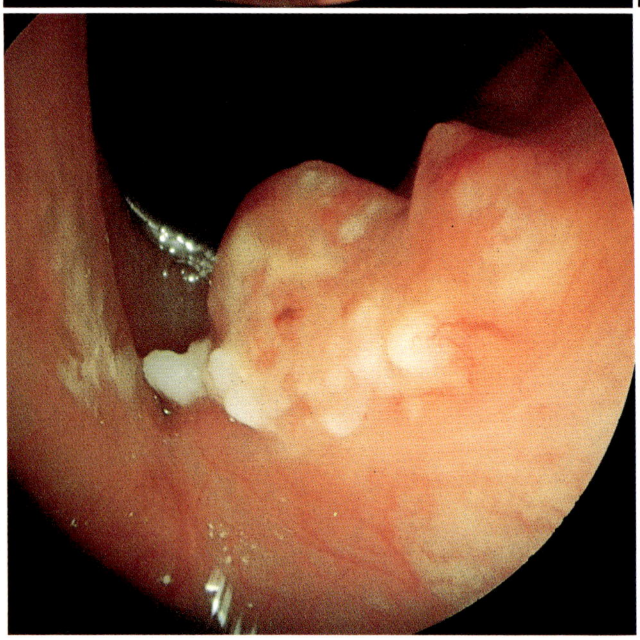

120°

FIG. 71. (Left column) This 50-year-old physician is a nonsmoker. Carcinoma of the right vocal cord is seen with the 0°, 70°, and 120° telescopes, which allow a multiperspective assessment.

FIG. 72. (Right column) This 64-year-old man is a cigarette smoker. He has carcinoma of the laryngeal vestibule. The 70° endoscope provides a view of the glottic level.

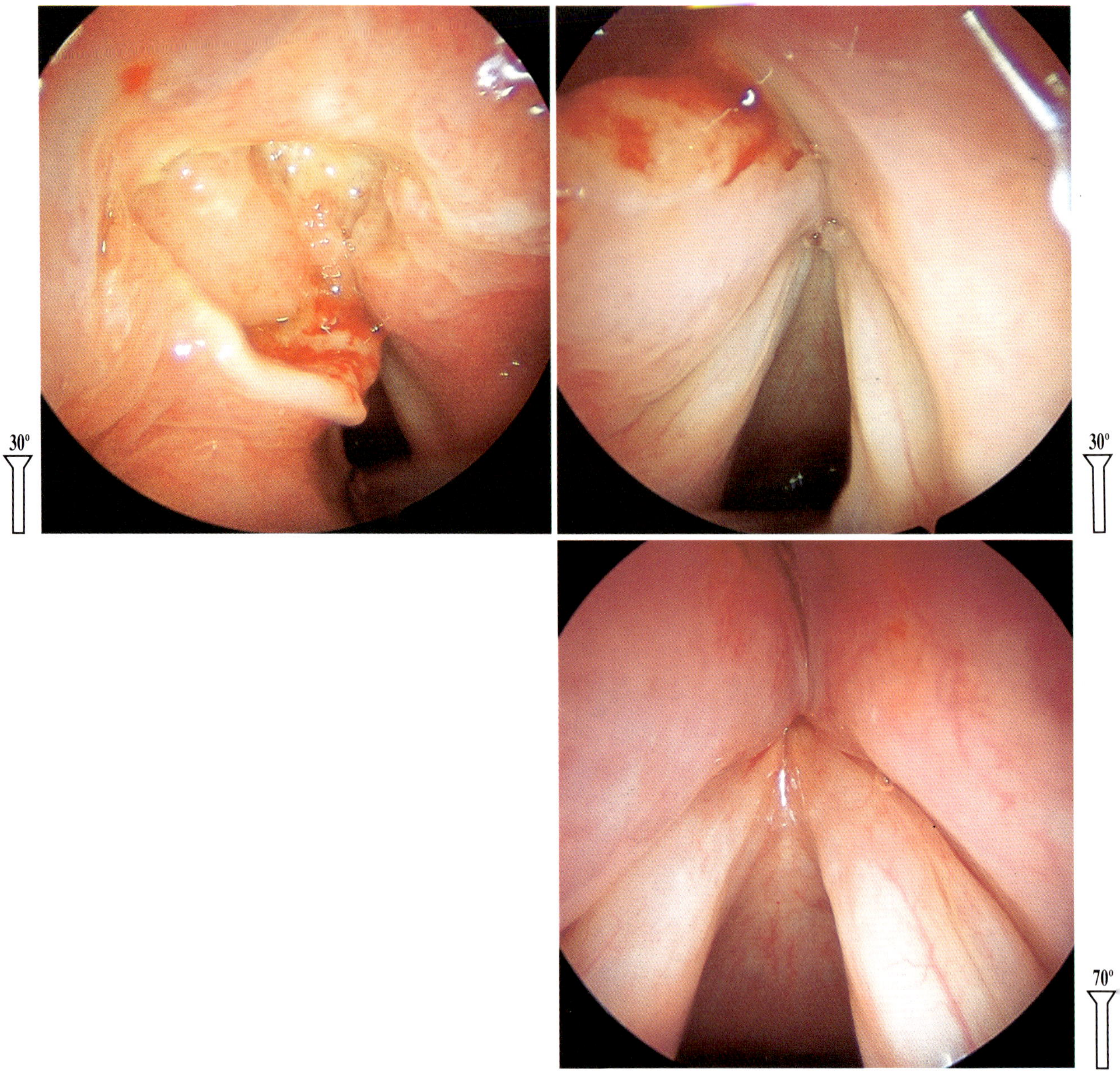

FIG. 73. This ulcerative, infiltrating supraglottic tumor occurred in a 51-year-old heavy smoker. Telescopes demonstrate invasion of the pre-epiglottic space, tumor margins, and the integrity of the glottic level.

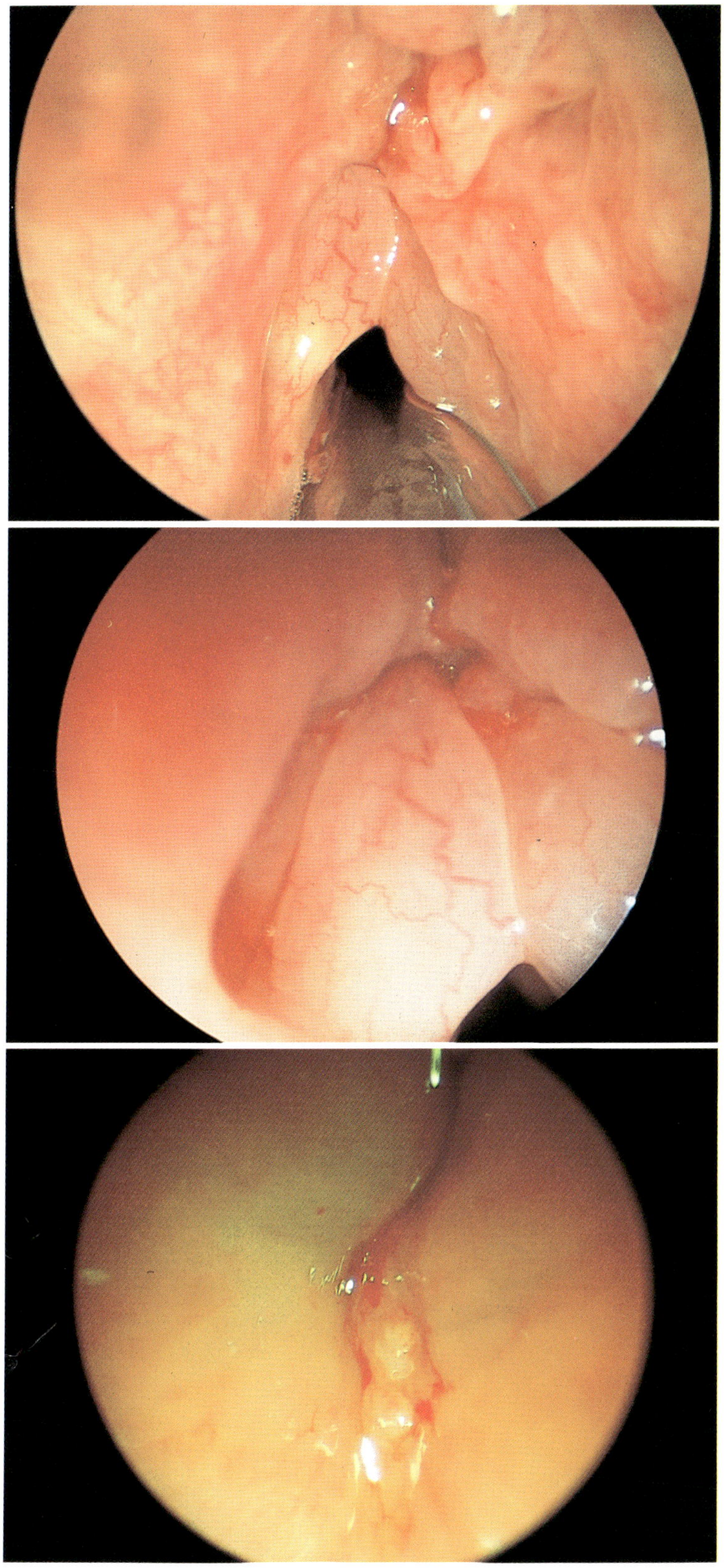

FIG. 74. Malignant tumor of the anterior aspect of the larynx occured in a 55-year-old heavy smoker. Telescopes allow assessment of tumor invasion at the supraglottis, glottis, and sub-glottis.

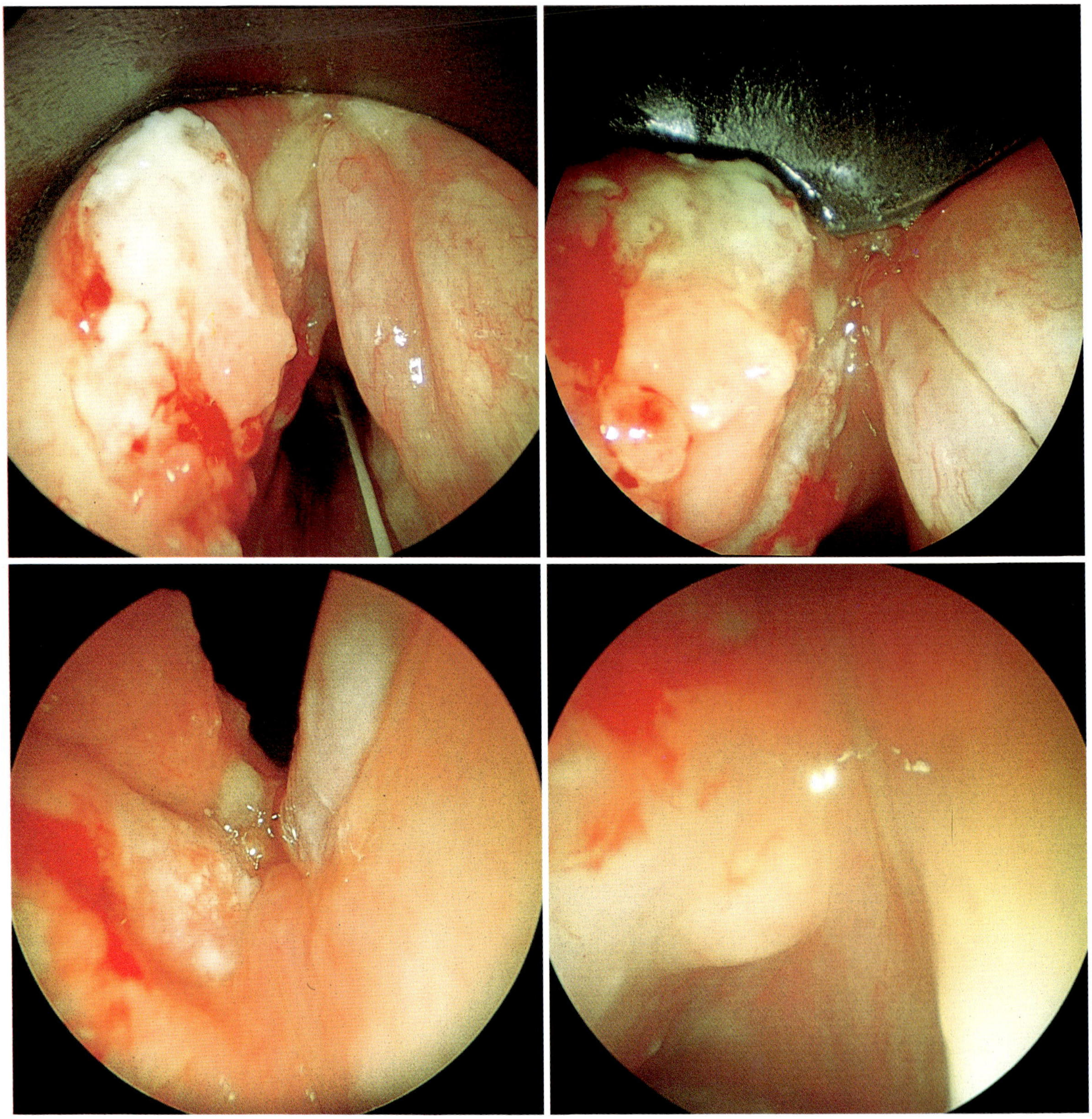

FIG. 75. This malignant tumor invades the left hemi-larynx in a 60-year-old patient.

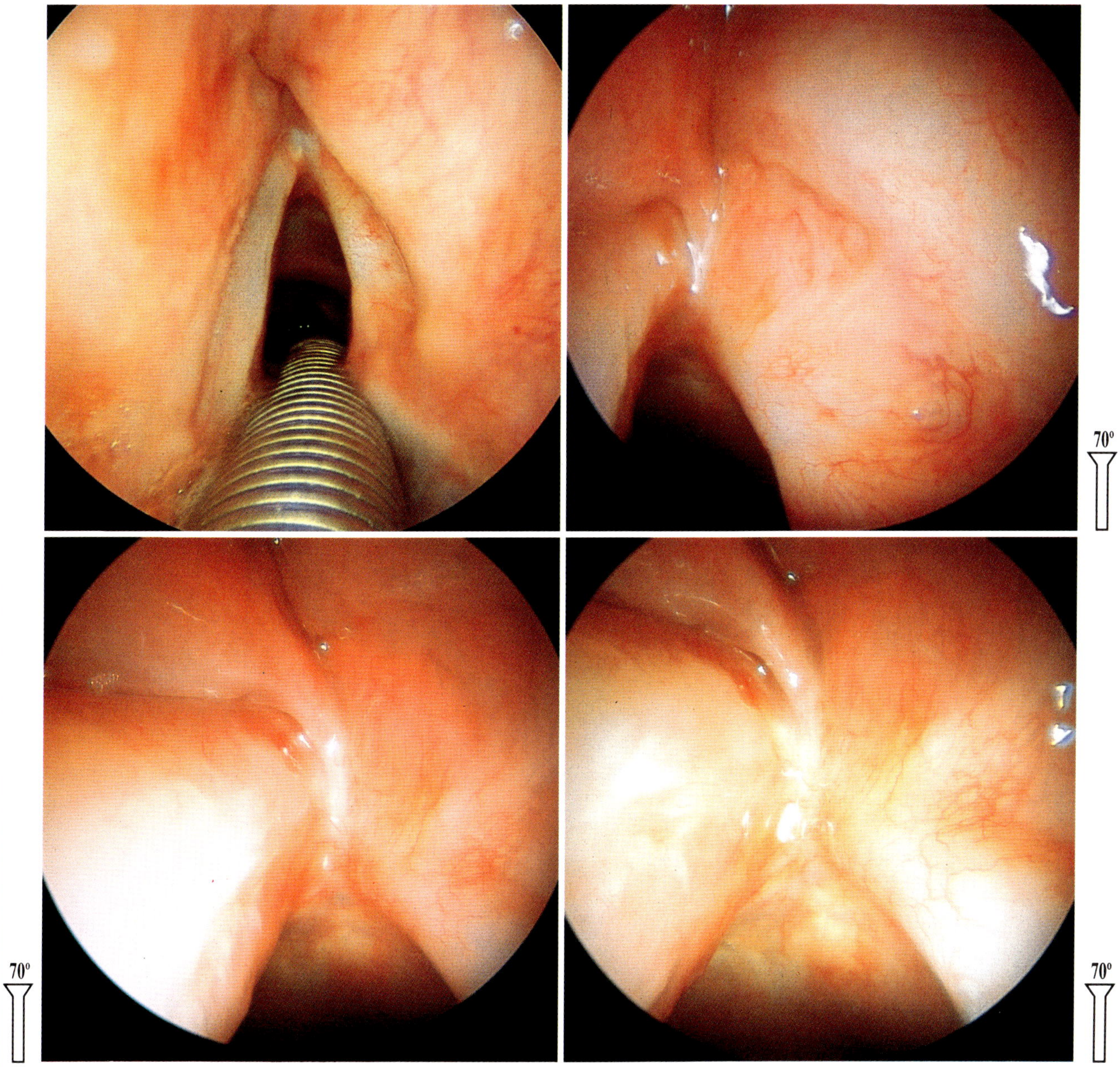

FIG. 76. These images relate to a 52-year-old male status-post right CO_2 laser cordectomy via an external approach one year ago. A suprastomal granuloma at the previous tracheostome necessitated endoscopic examination under general anesthesia. Besides the gap in the horizontal plane, there is another gap in the vertical axis between the superior surface of the left vocal cord and the superior limit of the conus elasticus and fibrotic tissue of the right side.

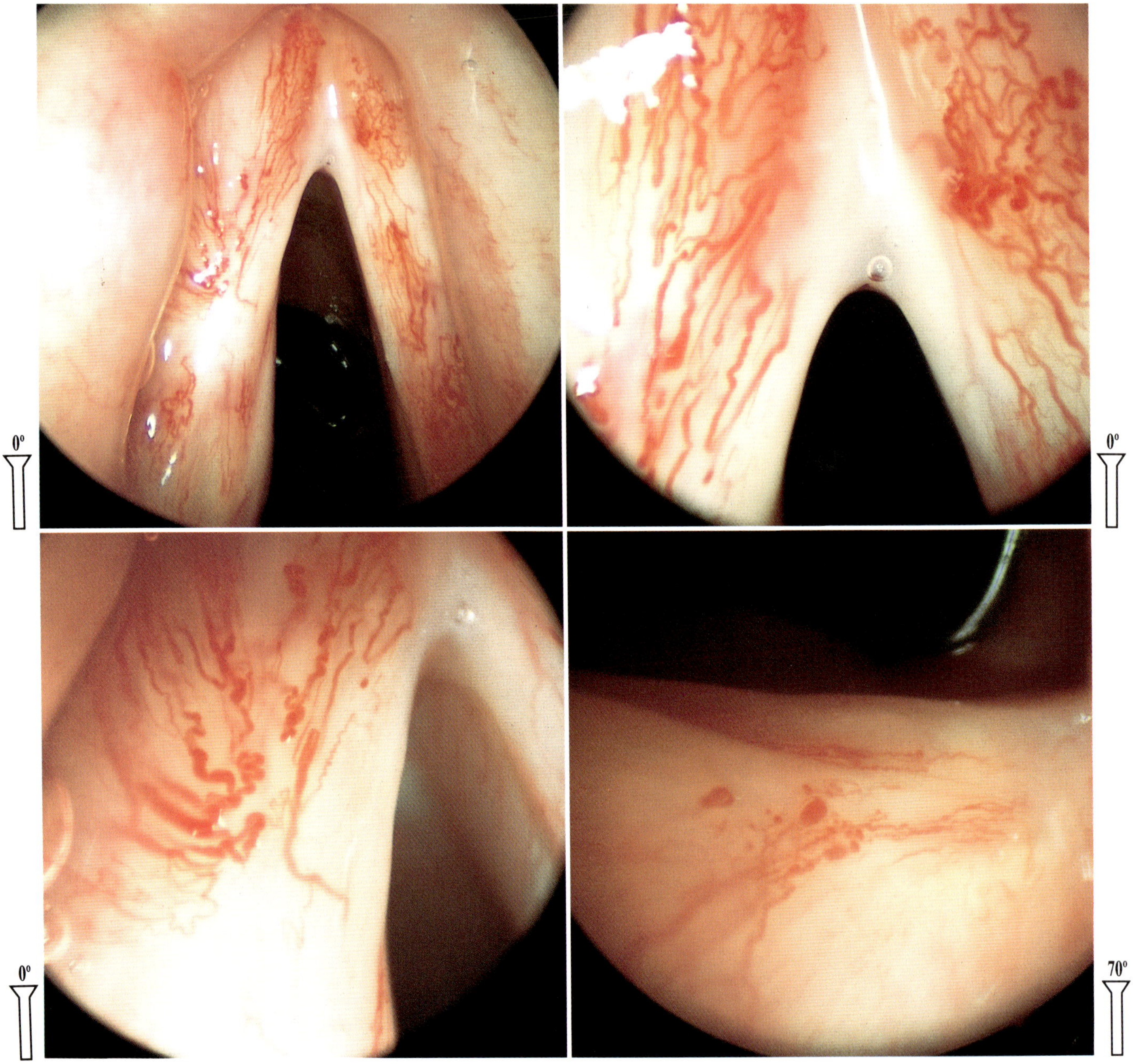

FIG. 77. This 65-year-old man's larynx was observed after 2 years of radiotherapy for a right vocal cord carcinoma. There is atrophic epithelium associated with deep alterations of the vascular pattern. The vocal cords are fibrotic and a synechia of the anterior commissure is evident.

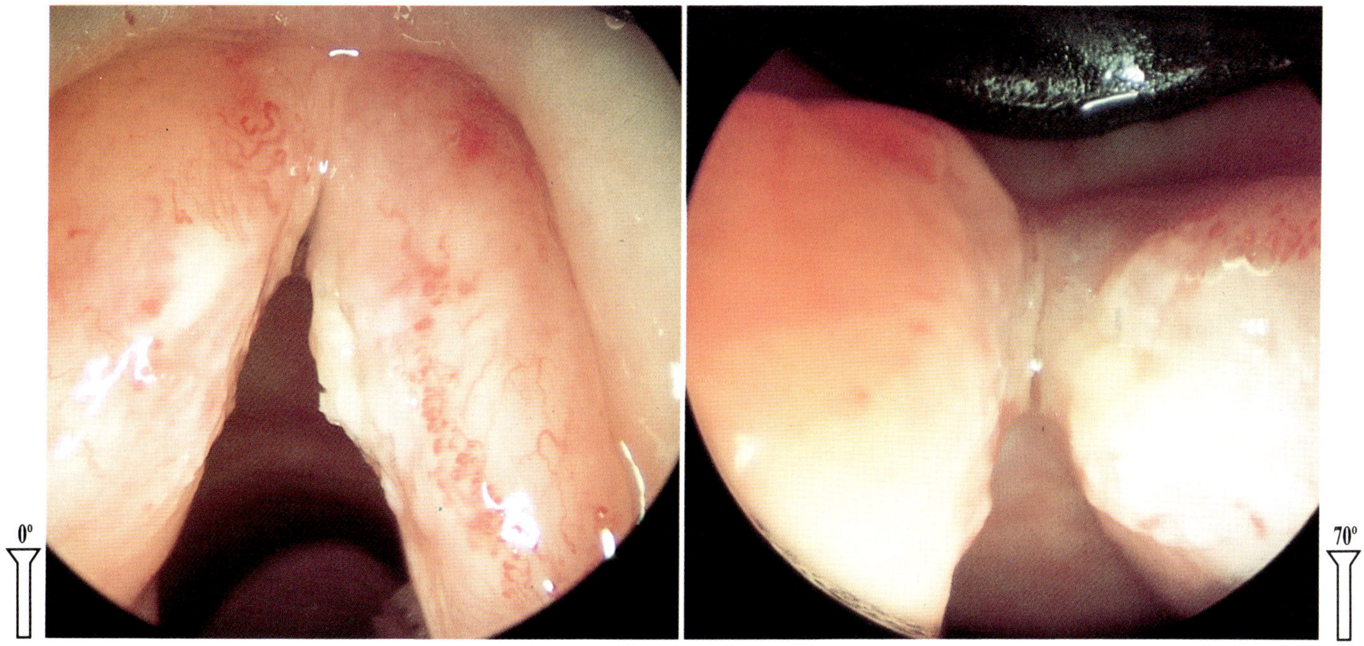

FIG. 78. This 55-year-old man's larynx was observed after 6 years of radiotherapy for a right vocal cord carcinoma.

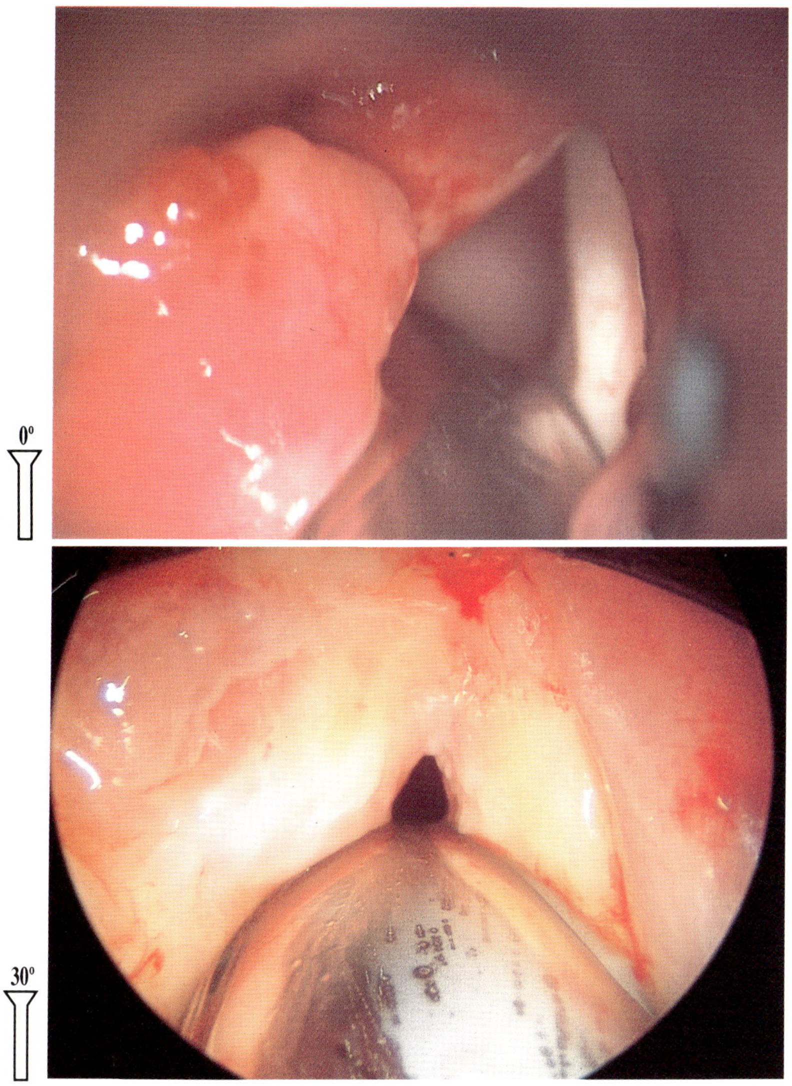

FIG. 79. These images document a malignant tumor of the left laryngeal vestibule in a 61-year-old female. The upper image was obtained before radiotherapy while the lower image was obtained 3 months after completion of radiation. The vocal cords are thickened, the mucosa atrophic, and there is a synechia noted at the anterior aspect of the glottis.

Part II: CEMS—Contact Endoscopy Associated with Microlaryngeal Surgery (Fig. 80)

Contact endoscopy allows an *in vivo* study of several cellular alterations in the vocal cord epithelium. A global assessment of the superficial layers of the epithelium is possible, from the normal to the abnormal, documenting different phases of the same disease.

Methylene blue was chosen as a vital staining agent because of its easy accessibility and widespread clinical use. However, the exact degree of penetration of the methylene blue into the epithelium remains to be determined. Other colorants such as Lugol's iodine or Waterman's blue ink, do not stain the vocal cord epithelium as well.

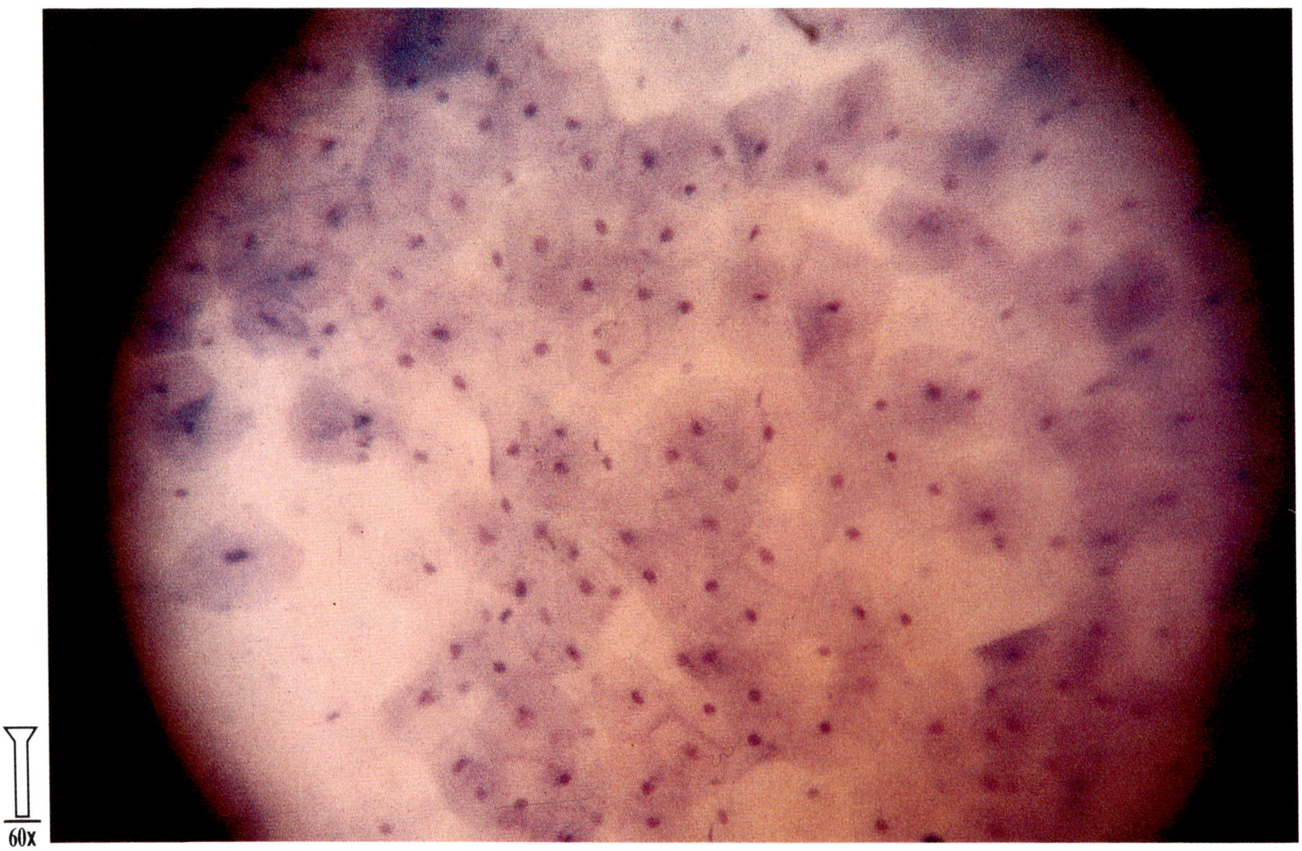

FIG. 80. Contact endoscopy of the vocal cord. The image was obtained by contact endoscopy (60×). Squamous epithelium is observed after methylene blue staining. The epithelium has a cellular population with a homogeneous pattern. The nucleus (dark blue) and the cytoplasm (light blue) show regular morphological characteristics: staining, shape, dimensions, and nucleus/cytoplasm ratio.

NORMAL PATTERN (Figs. 81–82)

A normal pattern of reference was defined based on contact endoscopy images obtained from the superior surface of the contralateral cord in 12 cases of polyps and 4 cases of vocal cord cysts. Moving the endoscope along the longitudinal axis of the vocal cord, the squamous epithelium is observed. The nuclei of its cells are identical in size and color. The cells are darkly stained, and the cytoplasm is light blue. The squamous cells have a polyhedric shape and are in continuity with each other, with a regular nucleus/cytoplasm ratio. The overall morphologic pattern is homogeneous.

Ciliated epithelium is also recognized with contact endoscopy. The dark blue nuclei are round, but the cytoplasmic limits of the cells are not as well defined as in the squamous epithelium. The filamentous structures displaced by the extreme end of the contact endoscope are composed of bundles of cilia.

Moving the contact endoscope laterally, the transition from squamous epithelium to the ciliated epithelium covering most of the endolarynx is observed. Variations in this transition are noticed. In some cases assessed as normal, the squamous epithelium, instead of being limited to the vocal edge, also covers the superior surface, although to a variable extent.

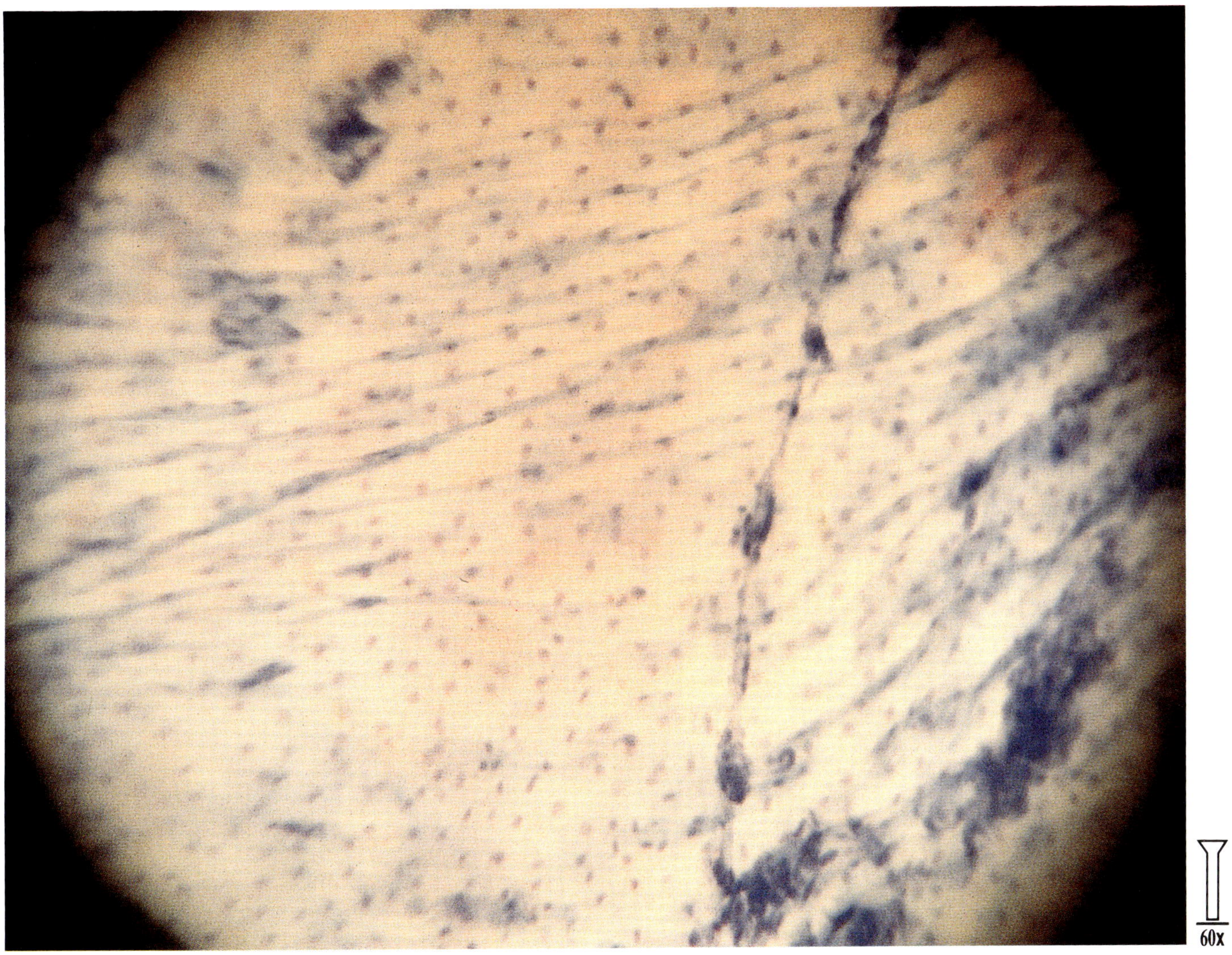

FIG. 81. Contact endoscopy of the vocal cord (60×). The cells have regular characteristics. The epithelial folds are evident at the vocal cord surface.

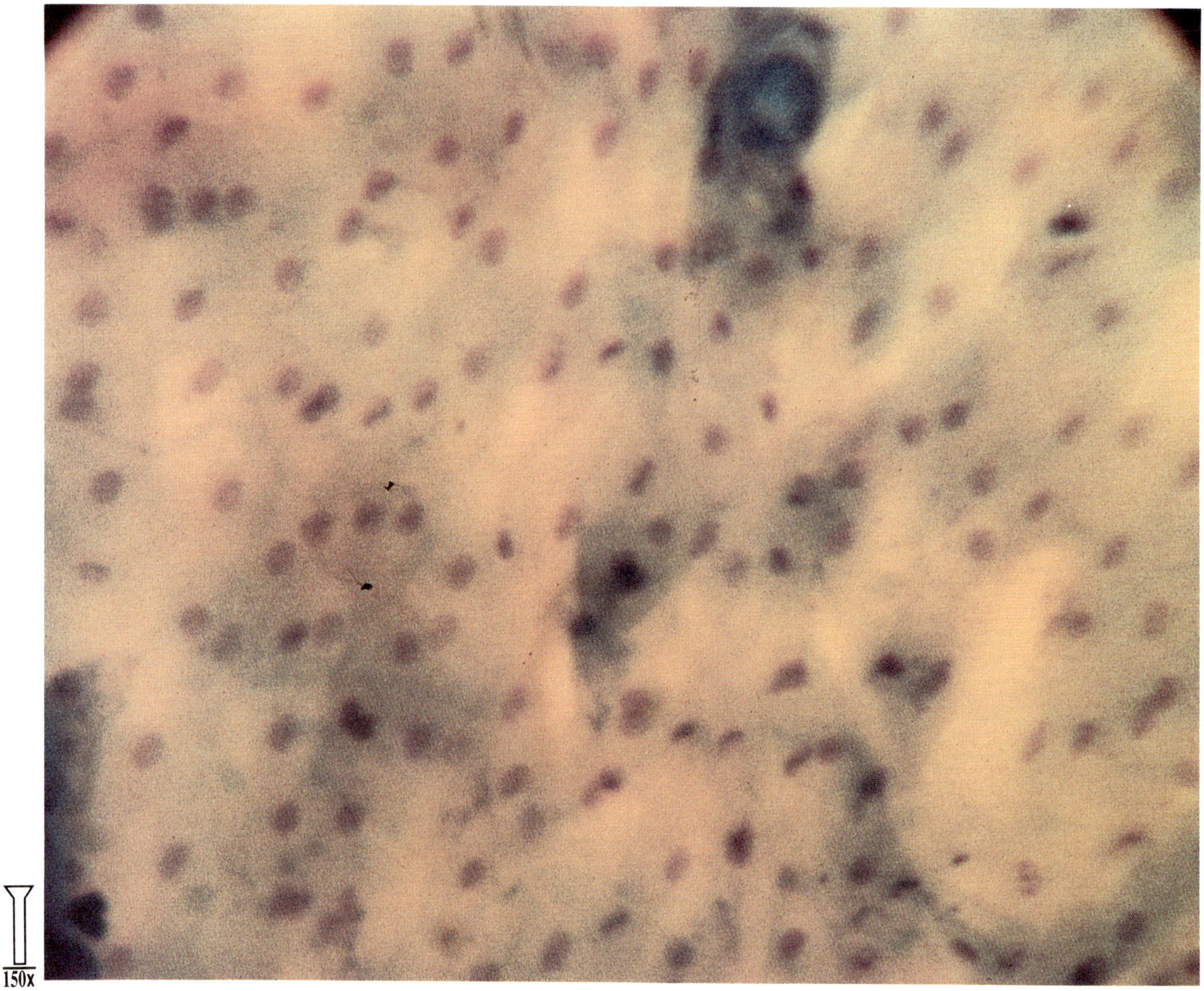

FIG. 82. Normal vocal cord squamous epithelium observed by contact endoscopy (×150). The higher magnification allows the nuclear characteristics to be seen in greater detail.

HISTOPATHOLOGY OF VOCAL EPITHELIUM (FIGS. 83–86)

To interpret contact endoscopy findings, contact videoendoscopic images were compared with histologic sections of biopsied or excised lesions, and laryngectomy specimens, fixed with 8 formalin immediately after surgery, were also analyzed. Fragments of the mucosa of vocal cords opposite the tumorous cords were collected for histology and electron microscopy preparation (scanning and transmission).

Because the vocal epithelium is exposed to external factors and because its cells have a limited life span, there is constant cell turnover. When external aggression is intensified, the epithelium reacts with hyperplasia or by producing a superficial layer of keratin, which creates the effect of a mechanical barrier. When localized, these plaques (hyperkeratosis) are visible by laryngoscopy.

Morphologic parameters used histopathologically to define a dysplastic cell are hyperchromatic nucleus, a nucleus of abnormally large or small dimensions, irregularity of the nuclear membrane, prominent nucleolus, increased number of mitoses, and superficial or abnormal mitoses. The presence of these alterations indicates intraepithelial neoplasia.

HISTOPATHOLOGY OF VOCAL EPITHELIUM (FIGS. 83–86)

To interpret contact endoscopy findings, contact videoendoscopic images were compared with histologic sections of biopsied or excised lesions, and laryngectomy specimens, fixed with 8 formalin immediately after surgery, were also analyzed. Fragments of the mucosa of vocal cords opposite the tumorous cords were collected for histology and electron microscopy preparation (scanning and transmission).

Because the vocal epithelium is exposed to external factors and because its cells have a limited life span, there is constant cell turnover. When external aggression is intensified, the epithelium reacts with hyperplasia or by producing a superficial layer of keratin, which creates the effect of a mechanical barrier. When localized, these plaques (hyperkeratosis) are visible by laryngoscopy.

Morphologic parameters used histopathologically to define a dysplastic cell are hyperchromatic nucleus, a nucleus of abnormally large or small dimensions, irregularity of the nuclear membrane, prominent nucleolus, increased number of mitoses, and superficial or abnormal mitoses. The presence of these alterations indicates intraepithelial neoplasia.

In pathology textbooks, the classification of degrees of dysplasia describes a series of alterations from dysplastic cells limited to the basal one-third of the epithelium (stage I) to stage III, in which all the epithelium is abnormal, also called carcinoma *in situ.* The intermediate stage, in which alterations exist in the basal two-thirds of the epithelium, is classified as stage II. When the integrity of the basement membrane is lost, invasive carcinoma is present. Contact videoendoscopy allows *in vivo* and *in situ* observation of the epithelium, but comparisons with histologic and electron microscopic studies of nontumorous vocal cords (obtained by laryngectomy) have shown that only the most superficial layers of the epithelium can be visualized. Since the contact endoscope is able to focus on subepithelial vessels, its inability to reveal the basal layers apparently results from a lack of penetration of methylene blue into the deeper epithelial layers.

Contact endoscopy images have shown that the transition between the two types of epithelium is not a smooth line. Islands of squamous metaplasia in the middle of ciliated epithelium have been identified. Histologic sections have shown that in certain metaplastic areas, squamous cells already existed under the ciliated epithelium. Further studies are needed to define the normal distribution of epithelium and the relationship of metaplasia to age and respiratory-irritant exposure.

Because of the dynamic migration of cells toward the surface of the epithelium, most pathology is ultimately expressed at the superficial layer and is then accessible to observation with contact endoscopy. Based on the study of 145 patients to date, we can delineate the following pathologic patterns.

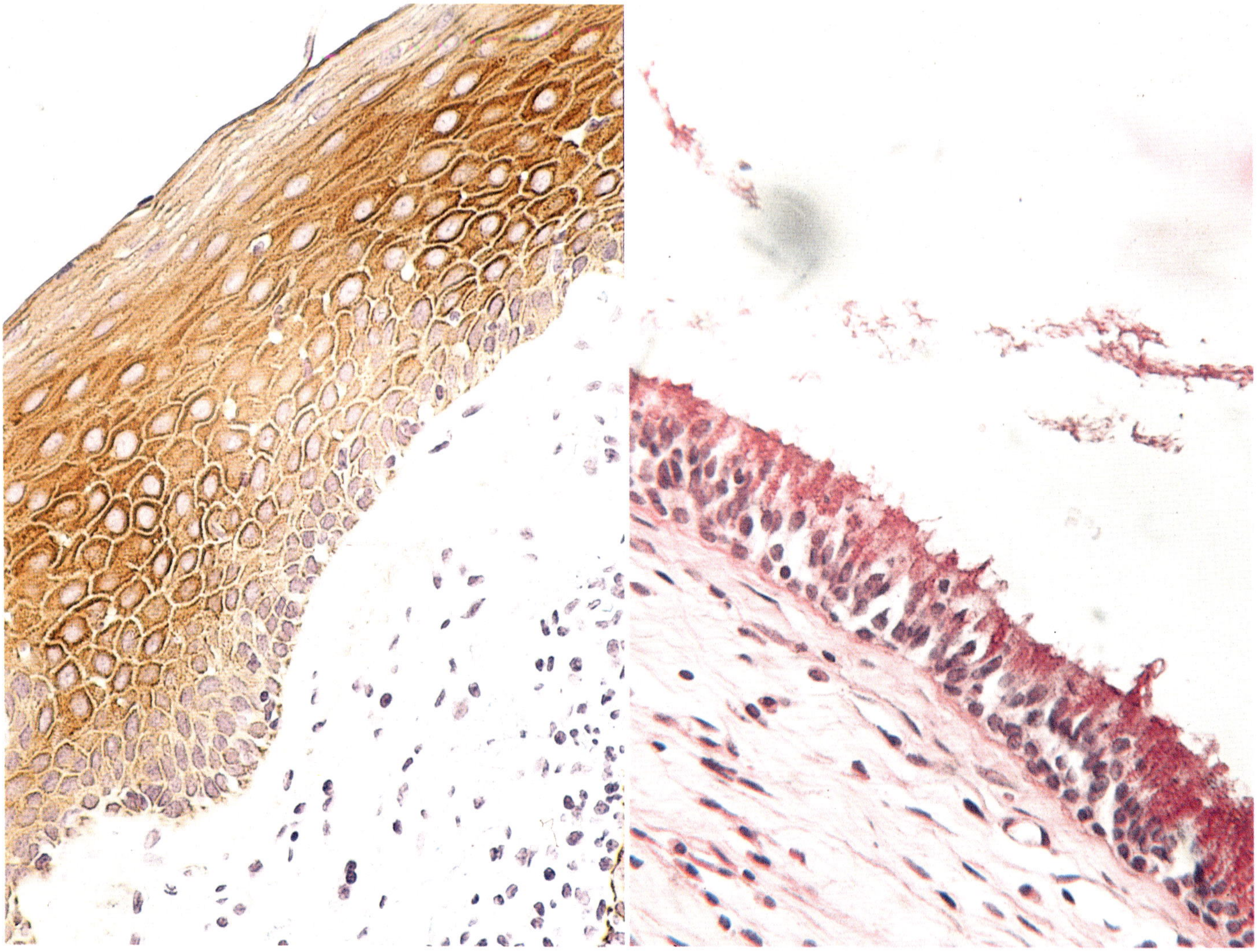

A B

FIG. 83. **A:** Squamous epithelium of the human vocal cord. Immunocytochemical anticytokeratin, 250×. **B:** Ciliated epithelium of the human vocal cord. H&E, 250×.

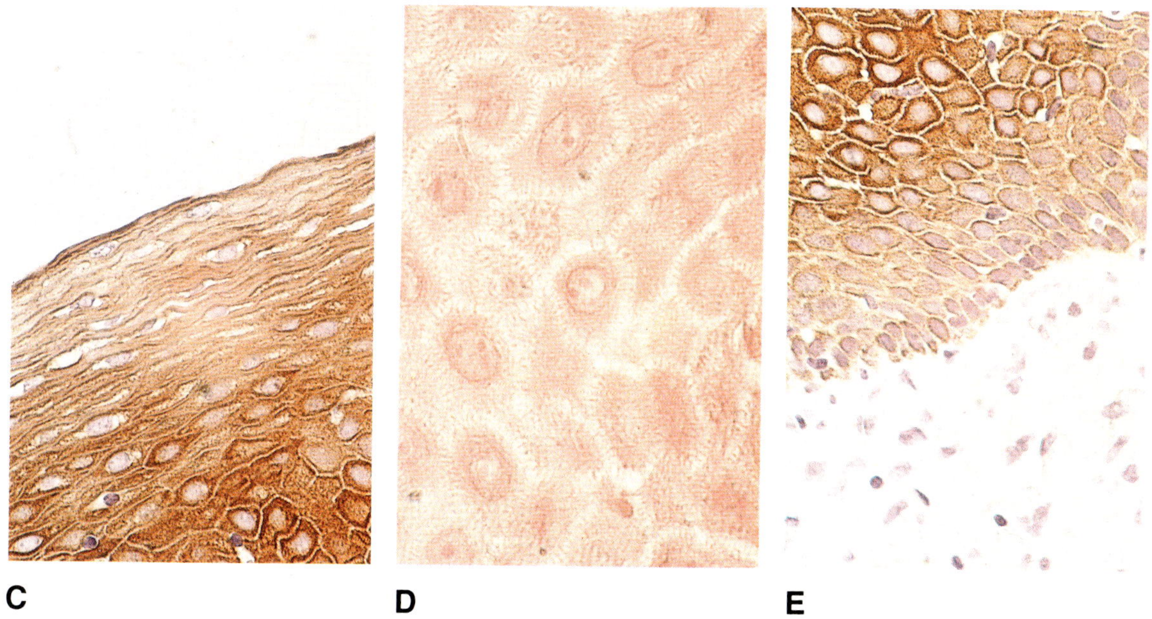

FIG. 83. *(continued).* **C:** Apical layers of the squamous epithelium. The typical flattened cells can be observed. Immunocytochemical anticytokeratin, 400×. **D:** Middle layers of the squamous epithelium. Desmosomes can be seen. H&E, 1000×. **E:** Basal layers of the squamous epithelium. In the germinative area of the epithelium, the cells have ovoid nuclei and scanty cytoplasm. Immunocytochemical anticytokeratin, 400×.

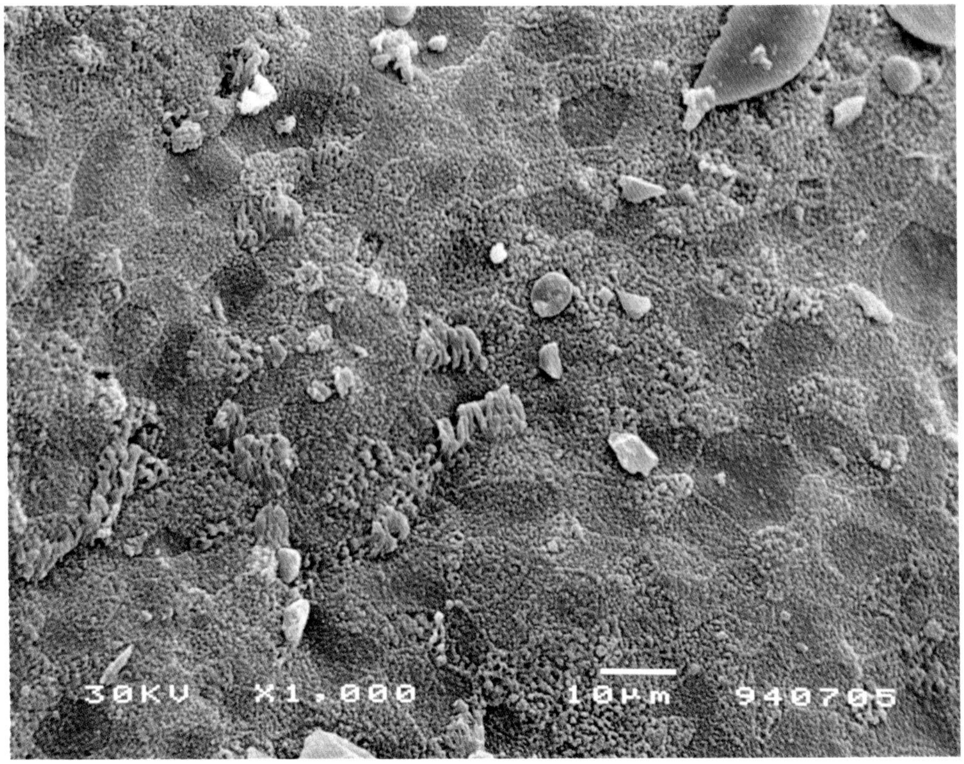
30KV X1,000
10µm
940705

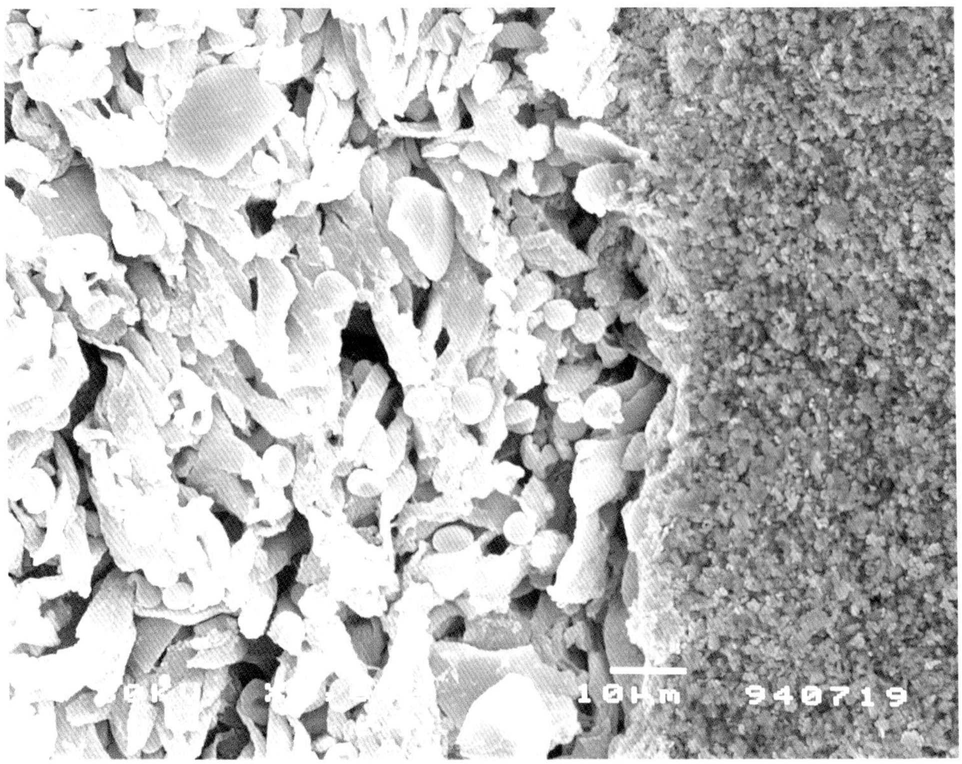
10µm
940719

FIG. 84. Scanning electron microscopy of vocal cord epithelium (1000×). Squamous cells covering the superior surface of the vocal cord can be observed. Islands of ciliated cells can also be distinguished among the squamous epithelium.

FIG. 85. Scanning electron microscopy of transition between ciliated epithelium (*left*) and squamous epithelium (*right*) 1000×.

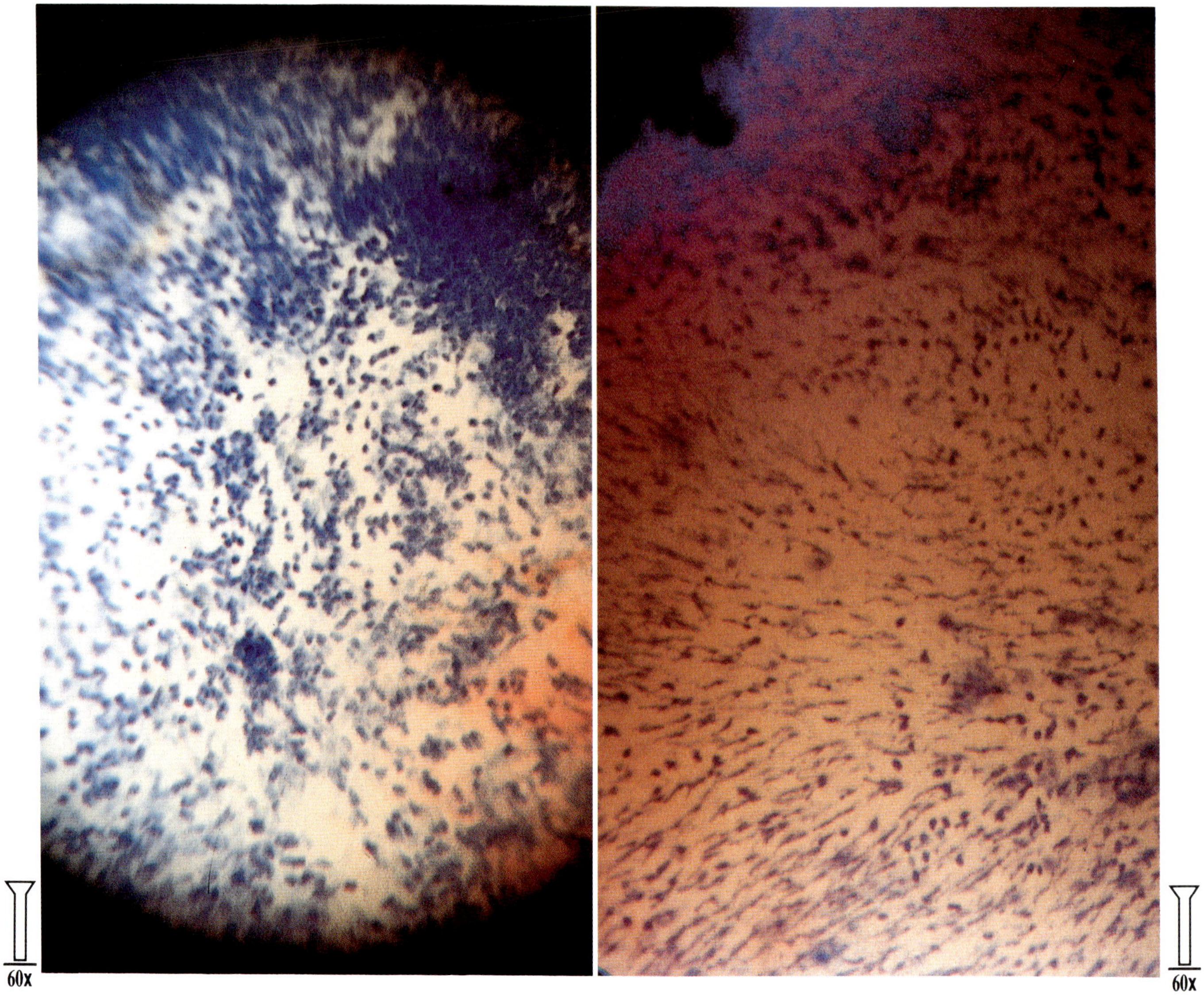

FIG. 86. Ciliated epithelium (*left* and *right*) observed by contact endoscopy 60×. The nuclei are dark blue. The filamentous structures are bundles of cilia that were displaced by the end of the telescope. The cytoplasmic limits of these cells are not as well defined as those of the squamous epithelium.

Chronic Laryngitis (87, 88)

In chronic laryngitis as observed by contact endoscopy, the epithelial pattern is homogeneous, but the nuclei are larger than normal and there is an increase in the nucleus/cytoplasm ratio. Squamous epithelium covers most of the superior surface of the vocal cord. The transition to ciliated epithelium is at the level of the ventricle. Because cell turnover is accelerated in the inflammatory reaction, it is possible to visualize immature cells at the surface that are similar to those usually present in the intermediate layers of normal epithelium.

In cases of Reinke's edema, normal epithelial cells with regular appearance and distribution, associated with slight changes suggestive of chronic laryngitis, were identified.

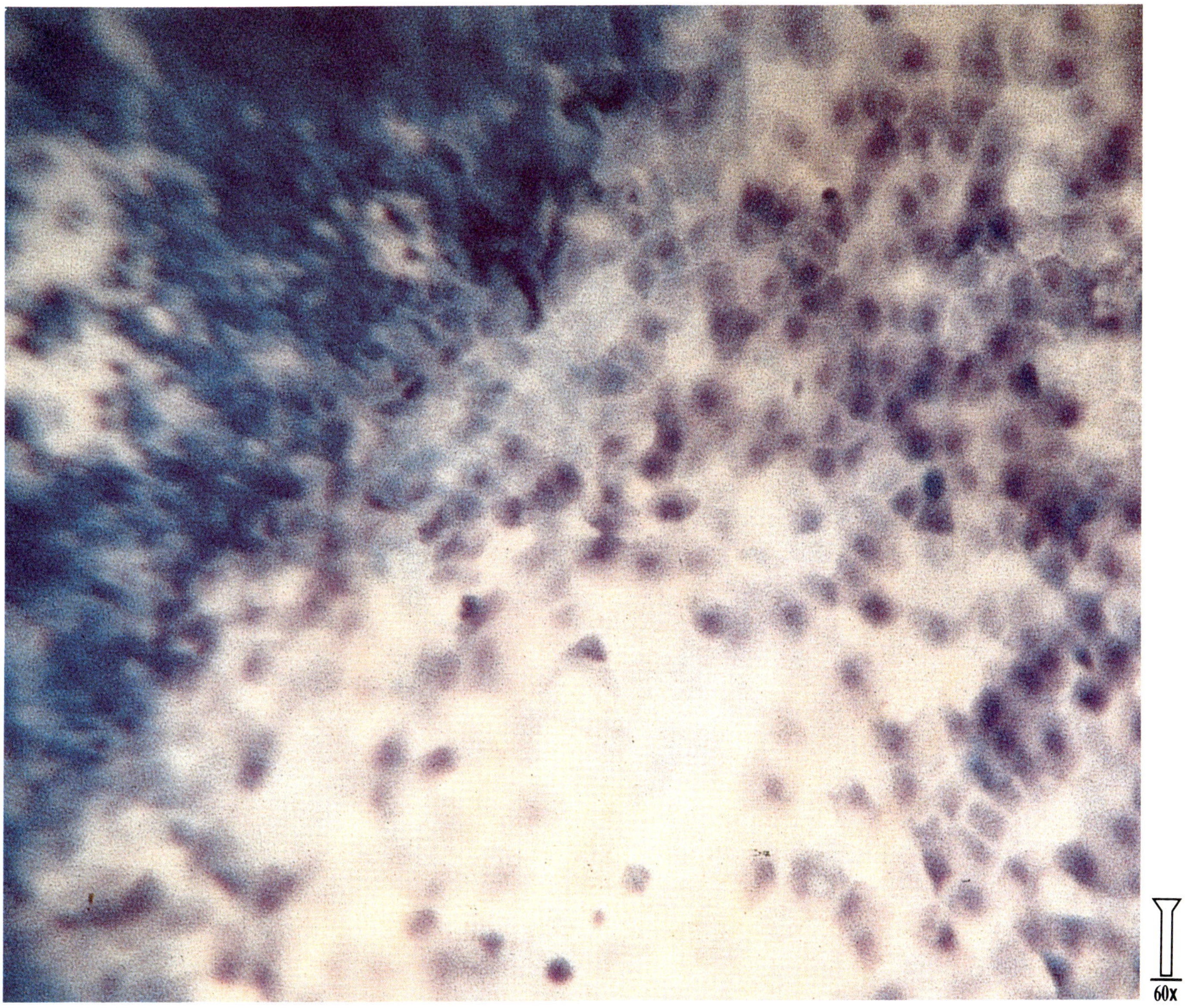

FIG. 87. Transition of ciliated/squamous epithelium observed by contact endoscopy 60×. The transition between ciliated epithelium and squamous epithelium is observed at the superior surface of the vocal cord near the floor of the Morgagni ventricle. The nuclei of the squamous epithelium are enlarged, suggesting chronic inflammation.

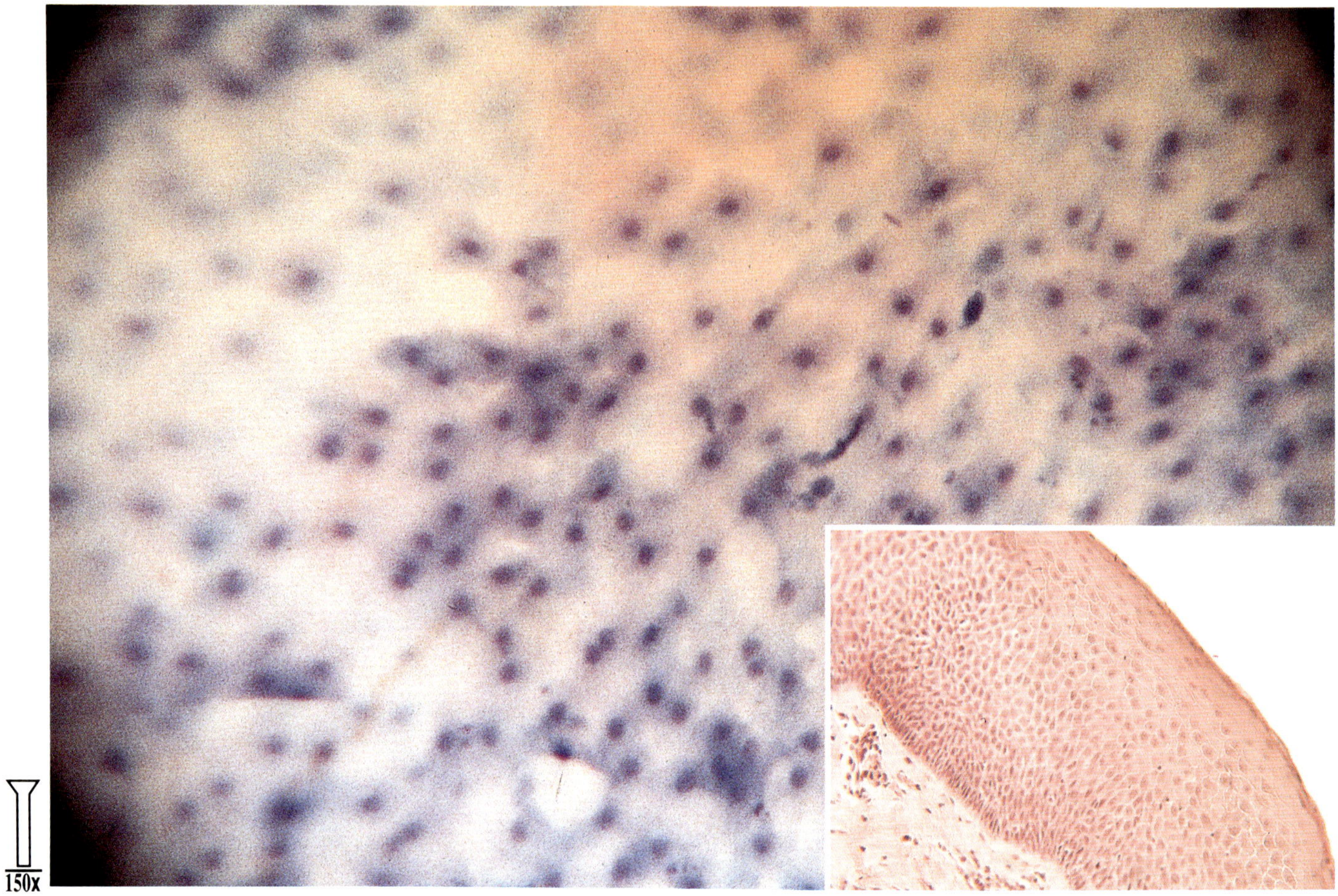

FIG. 88. Chronic laryngitis (contact endoscopy, 150×). This pathologic pattern is characterized by nuclei with increased dimensions and a high nucleus/cytoplasm ratio. Staining, limits, and shape still have regular characteristics with a homogeneous distribution.
FIG. 88A. Histologic section (Weigert, 250×) of chronic laryngitis. There is epithelial hyperplasia with an increased number of cellular layers. At the basal layer, there is hyperplasia, but there are no atypical cells.

Keratosis (Figs. 89,90)

Keratosis is easily documented with CEMS because it is an alteration at the surface of the epithelium. Contact endoscopy shows distinct stages of keratinization, which can occur simultaneously. In the initial stages of keratinization, isolated, light blue cells without nuclei are observed. More advanced stages show groups of cells without nuclei, but distinct cells can still be identified. Finally, individual cells cannot be distinguished, and only large areas of amorphous or laminar structures are visible. Initial stages of keratosis detected by contact endoscopy are not detected by office endoscopic techniques, microlaryngoscopy, or even using telescopes.

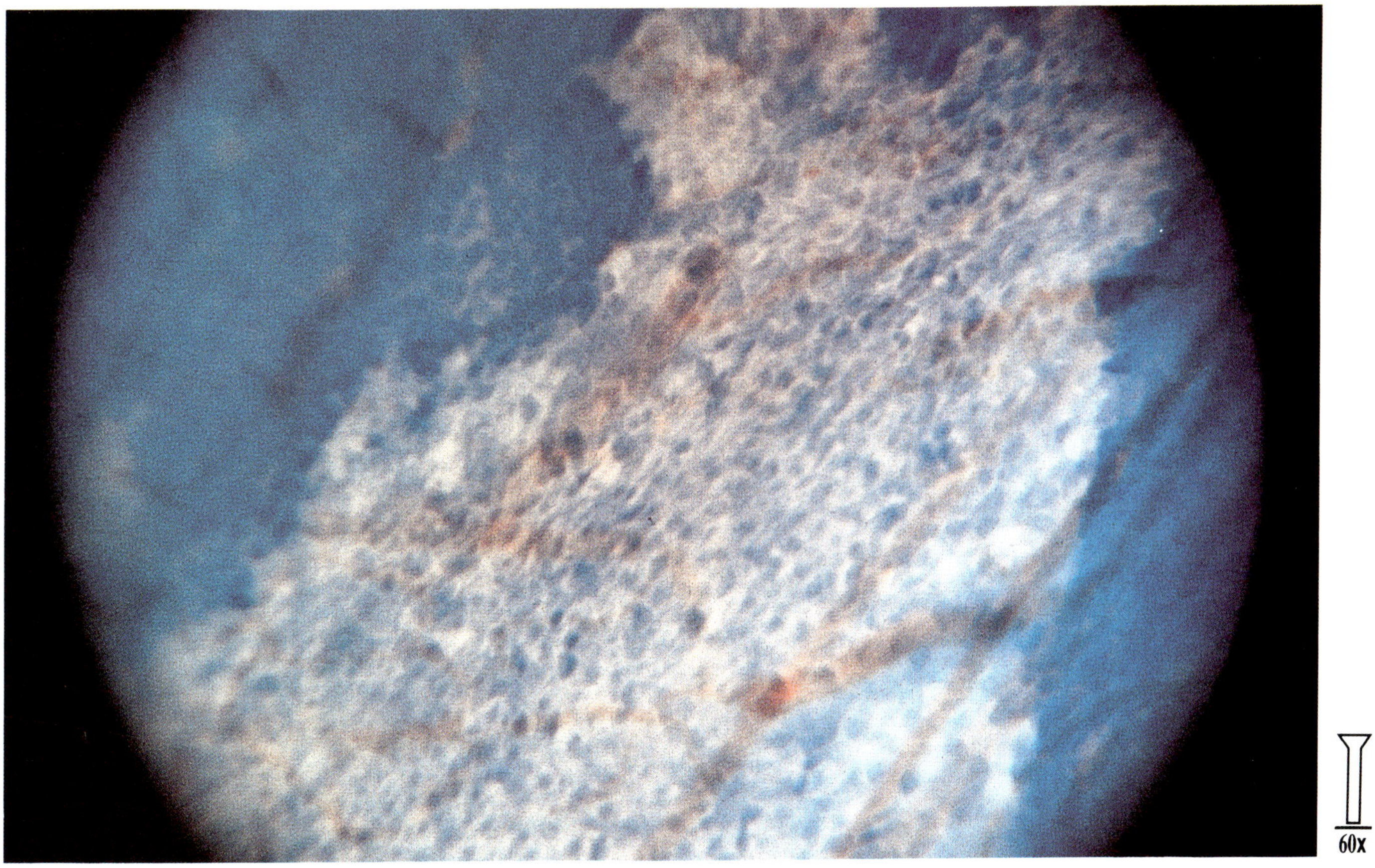

FIG. 89. Keratosis (contact endoscopy, 60×). Areas with different degrees of keratinization can be identified. Keratotic plaques consist of keratin agglomerates. The cellular limits of the squamous cells cannot be identified in the advanced stage.

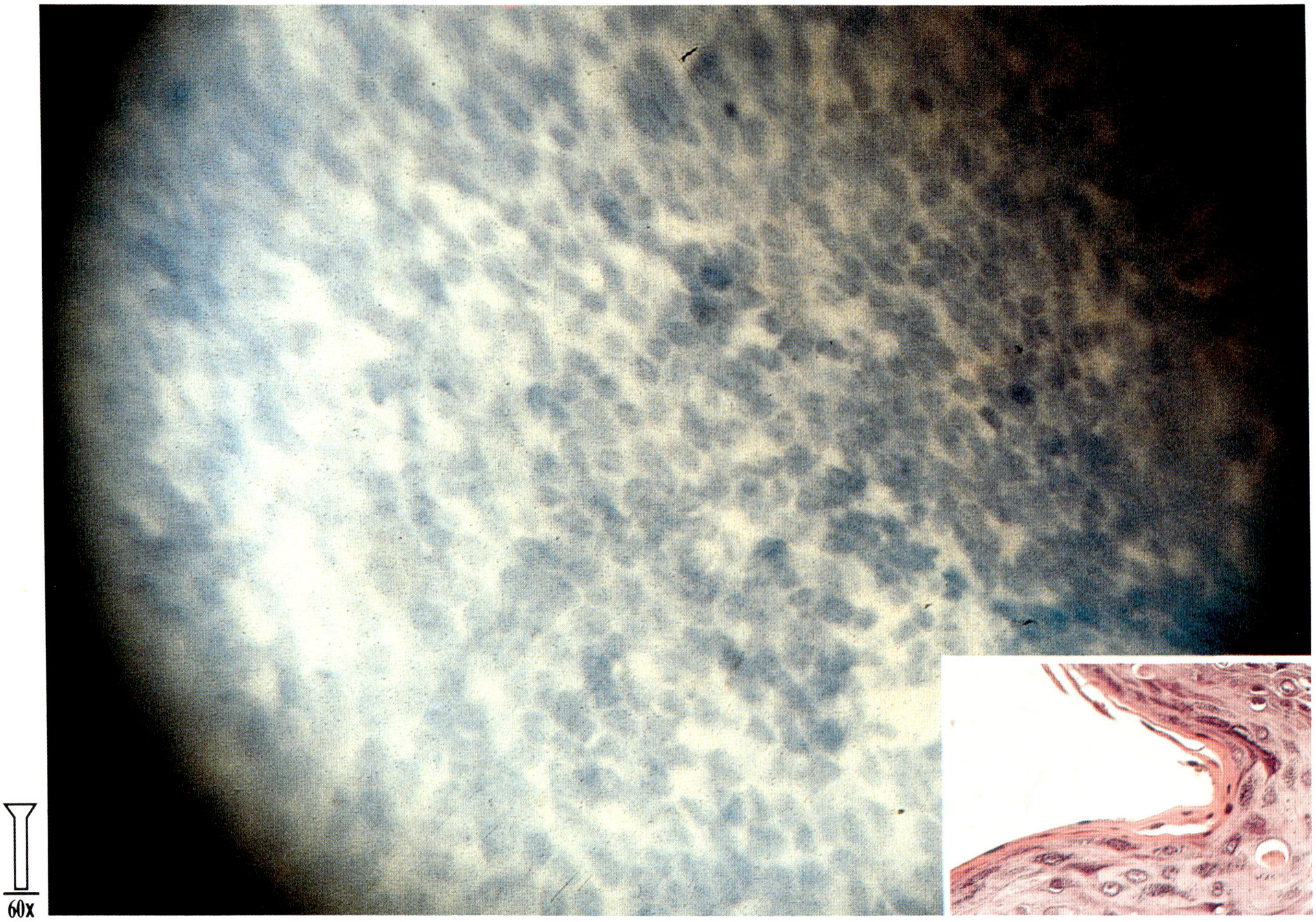

FIG. 90. Keratosis (contact endoscopy, 60×). In this early stage of keratinization individual cells without nuclei are still indentified.
FIG. 90A. Histologic section (Mallory, 400×) of keratosis. There is epithelial hyperplasia with no atypical cells. Keratosis is visible on the surface.

Dysplasia (Fig. 91)

In some cases of leukoplakias, apart from keratosis, other types and degrees of abnormalities can be identified, such as heterogeneity of cell population with nuclei of different color, size, and shape. The variety of images obtained is consistent with the macroscopic concept of leukoplakia, integrating different pathologic alterations such as hyperkeratosis, dysplasia, or neoplasia (15,19,20,34,36, 41,42).

Pathologic examination has shown that superficial assessment of dysplasia with contact endoscopy does not allow detection of stage I dysplasia. However, those stages of dysplasia that involve the superficial layers are accessible to the contact endoscope. Thus, the more cell abnormalities detectable with contact videoendoscopy, the more severe the dysplasia.

Most of the cellular alterations required for the diagnosis of dysplasia can be documented by contact endoscopy, including the presence of severe nuclear abnormalities (in size, hyperchromasia, and shape), alterations of the nucleus/cytoplasm ratio, dyskaryosis, dyschromasia, and the presence of mitoses and anisokaryosis (characterized by the presence of nuclei of various sizes in a single optical field). Different stages of the disease can be identified with the contact endoscope on a superficial level.

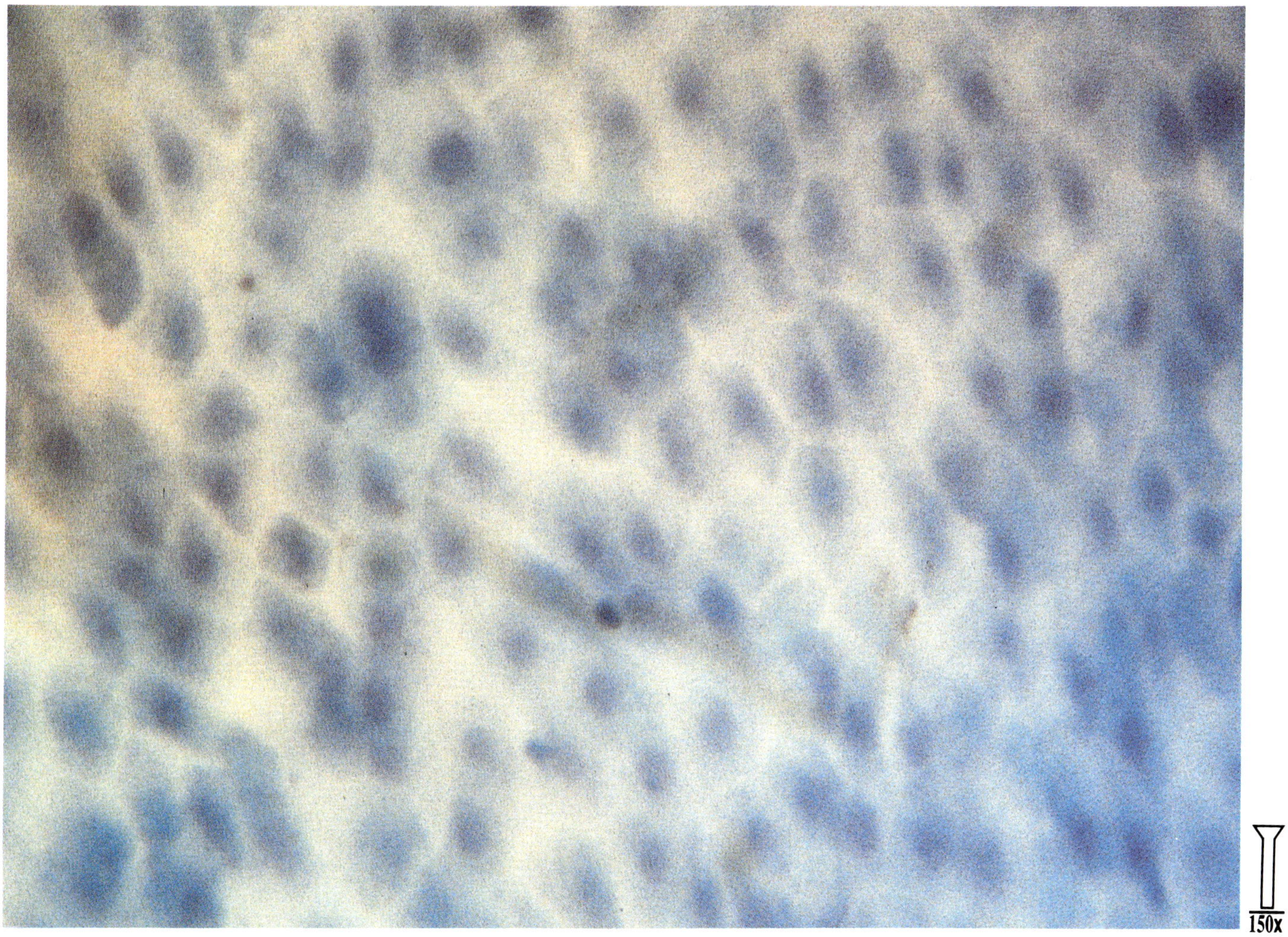

FIG. 91. Dysplasia (contact endoscopy, 150×). In this image the general pattern of the superficial layers of the epithelium is heterogeneous. The nuclei have increased diminsions and irregular staining.

Malignant Tumor (Figs. 92,93)

In carcinomas, contact videoendoscopic examination shows the irregularity of cell distribution and the extreme heterogeneity of cells, with nuclei of different staining properties, sizes, and shapes. The nucleus/cytoplasm ratio is very irregular. Nuclear inclusion bodies, prominent nucleoli, and mitoses are also evident.

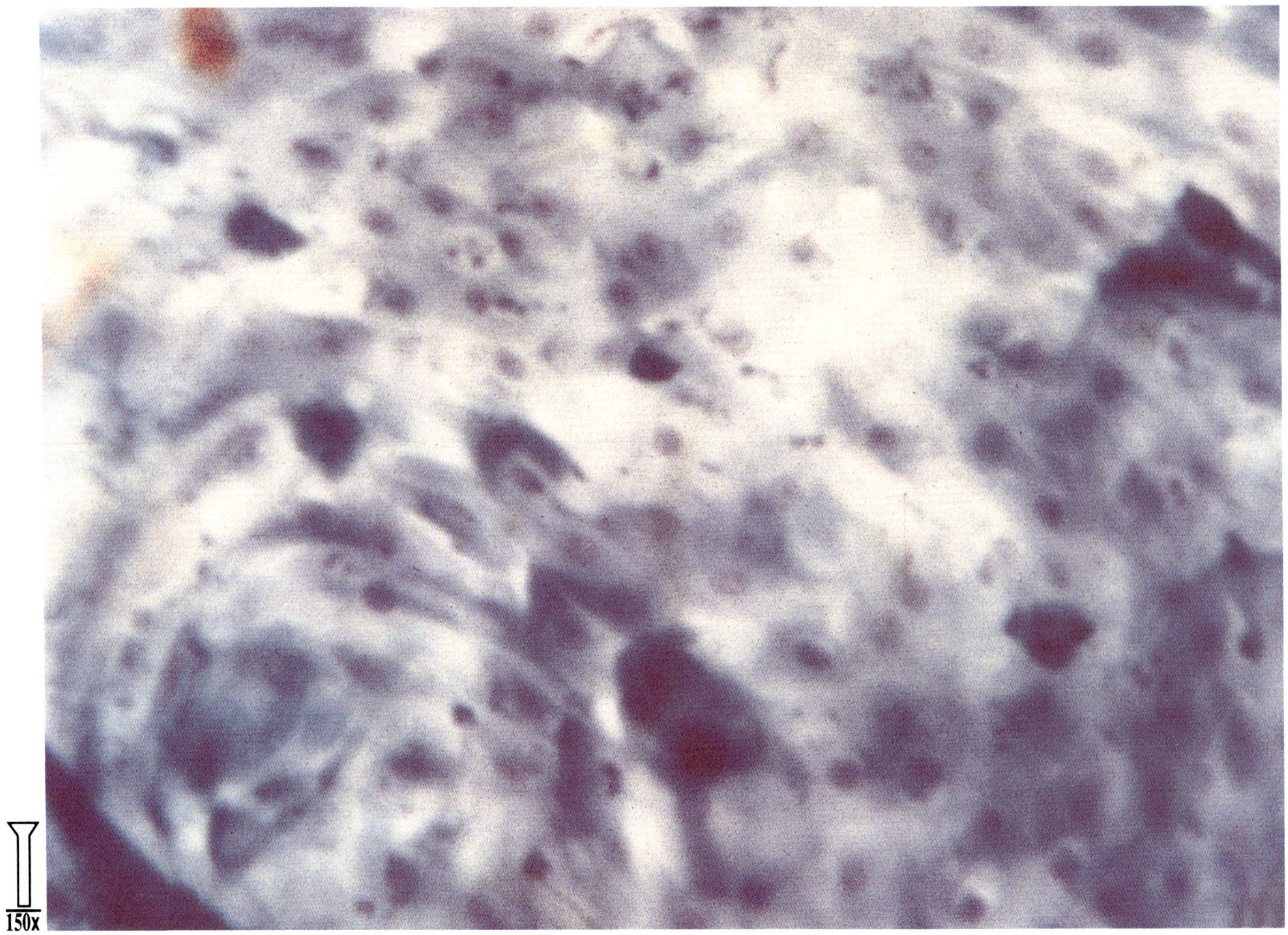

FIG. 92. Tumor (contact endoscopy, 150×). The cell pattern is very irregular with nuclei with extensive abnormalities—size, shape, limits, staining, and nucleus/cytoplasmic ratio.

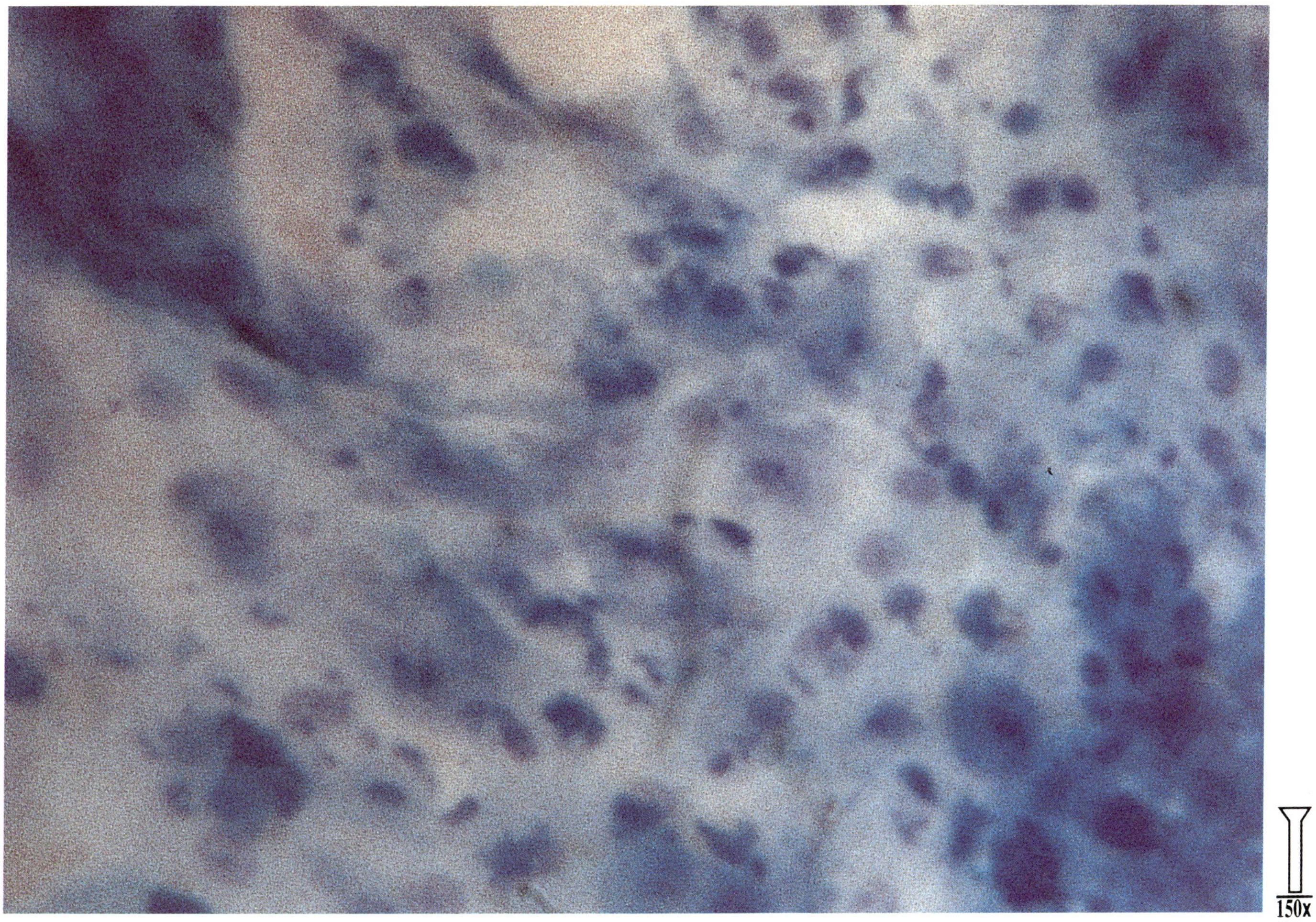

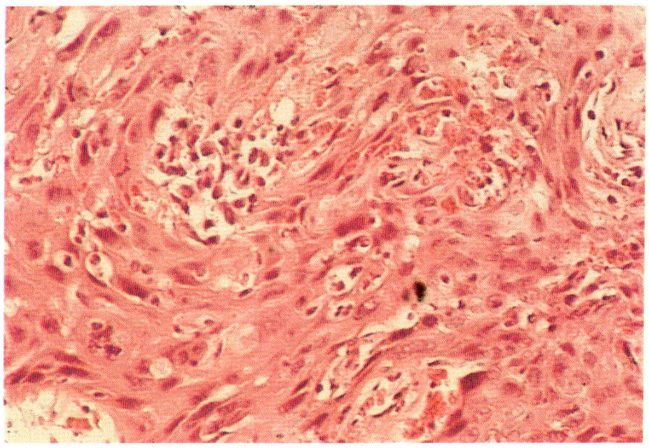

FIG. 93. Tumor (contact endoscopy, 150×). Some characteristic nuclear anomalies can be noticed in a single optical field, dyschromasia and anisokaryosis. Polymorphonuclear infiltrates are also present, associated with the cellular heterogeneity of the tumor.
FIG. 93A. Carcinoma with atypical cell and inflammatory infiltrate. H&E, 250×.

Papillomatosis/Papilloma (Figs. 94, 95)

In papillomatosis, contact endoscopy allows the visualization of multiple papillae covered by squamous epithelium. Each papilla has a vessel along a central axis. Between the papillae, there is a spiral arrangement of keratin; the ability to visualize the vascular structures is reduced with increasing keratosis.

In adult papillomas, koilocytes (ballooned cells) are observed. These cells have a vacuolated cytoplasm, with the nucleus displaced to the periphery, often molded into a crescent by the compression of the cytoplasmic vacuole. In the histologic sections, multilobulated leukocytes (polymorphonuclear cells) were also identified. Differences between juvenile papillomatosis and adult papilloma can be seen in the degree of keratosis and the presence of koilocytes and immature cells.

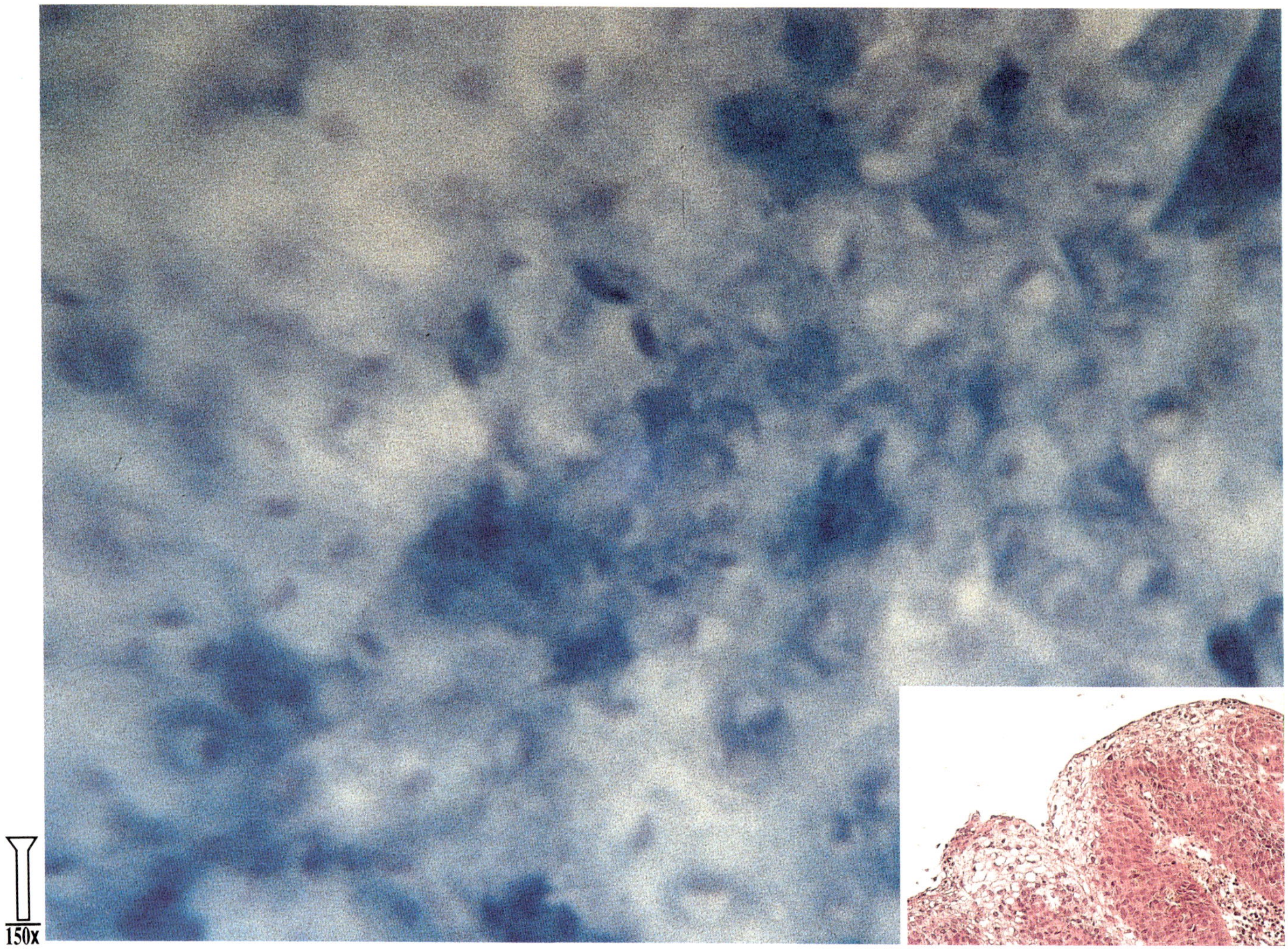

FIG. 94. Papilloma (contact endoscopy, 150×). Ballooned cells are visible. A cytoplasmic vacuole pushes the nucleus to the periphery of the cell. Inflammatory cells, with large but regular nuclei, are also present. Sometimes it is possible to identify polymorphonuclear infiltrates in the epithelium.

FIG. 94A. Histologic section of papilloma. The papillary epithelial structure is evident. The squamous hyperplastic epithelium has ballooned cells (koilocytes). The number of mitoses is increased but there are no atypical cells. Inflammatory infiltration of the mucosa is evident. H&E, 250×.

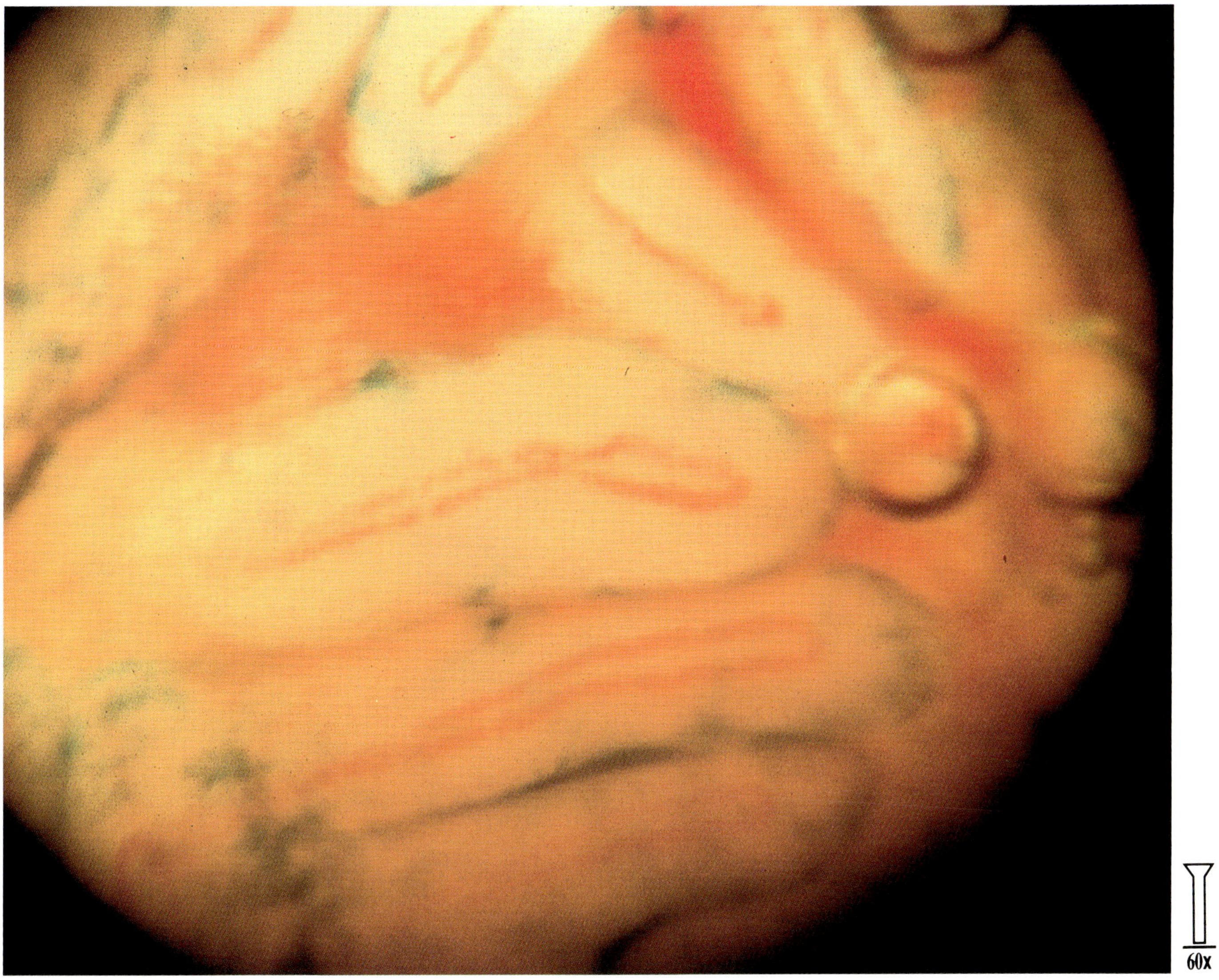

FIG. 95. Papillomatosis (contact endoscopy, 60×). A papillary arrangement with a vascular axis can be observed.

Microvascular Patterns (Figs. 96–99)

Contact videoendoscopy allows the *in vivo* observation of the vocal cord vessels, making it possible to document their pattern of distribution and circulatory dynamics. Longitudinal vessels of different calibers are linked by a network of anastomoses with distinct orientations. These anastomoses function intermittently, as can be seen observing the blood flow. Also, the vessels are arranged in different planes with anastomoses between them. The blood may flow in different directions even in adjacent vessels situated in the same plane. Circulating red cells can be observed using 150× magnification.

In different pathologic situations, there are distinct vascularization patterns. Abnormalities that have been documented include reinforcement of the vascular network with exuberant anastomosis, vascular ectasias, thrombosed vessels, accumulation of erythrocytes inside atypical vessels, vessels with diminished circulation, increased space between the vessels, vessels with a spiral appearance, papillary vessels, corkscrew vessels, and atypical capillaries.

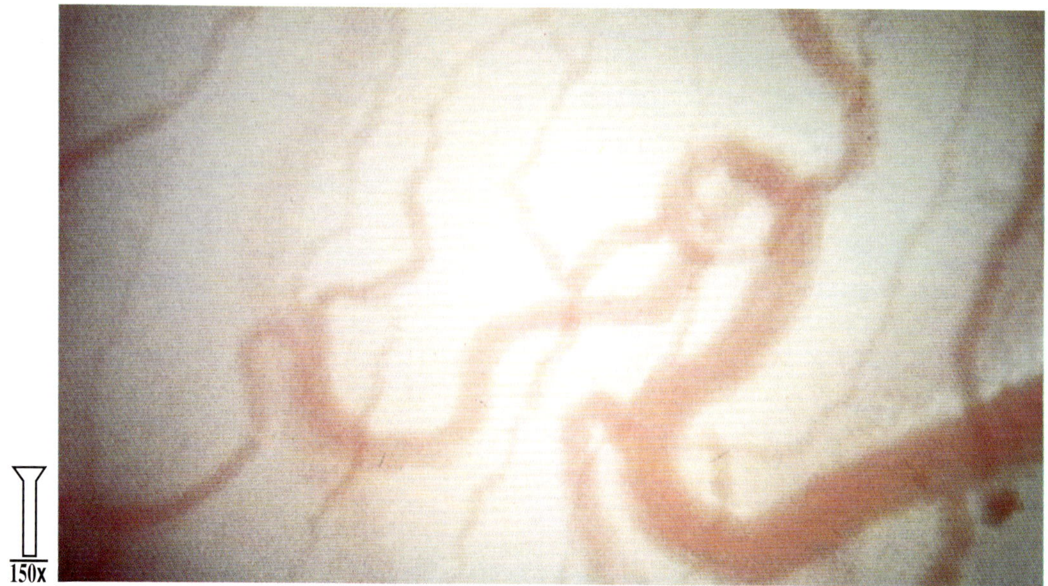
150x

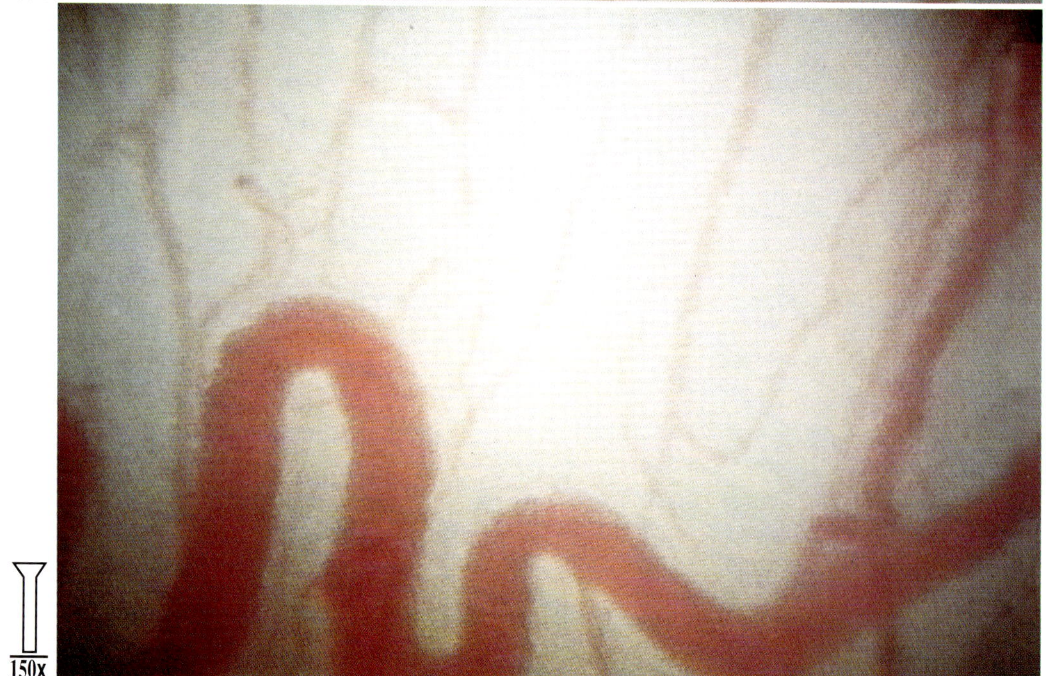
150x

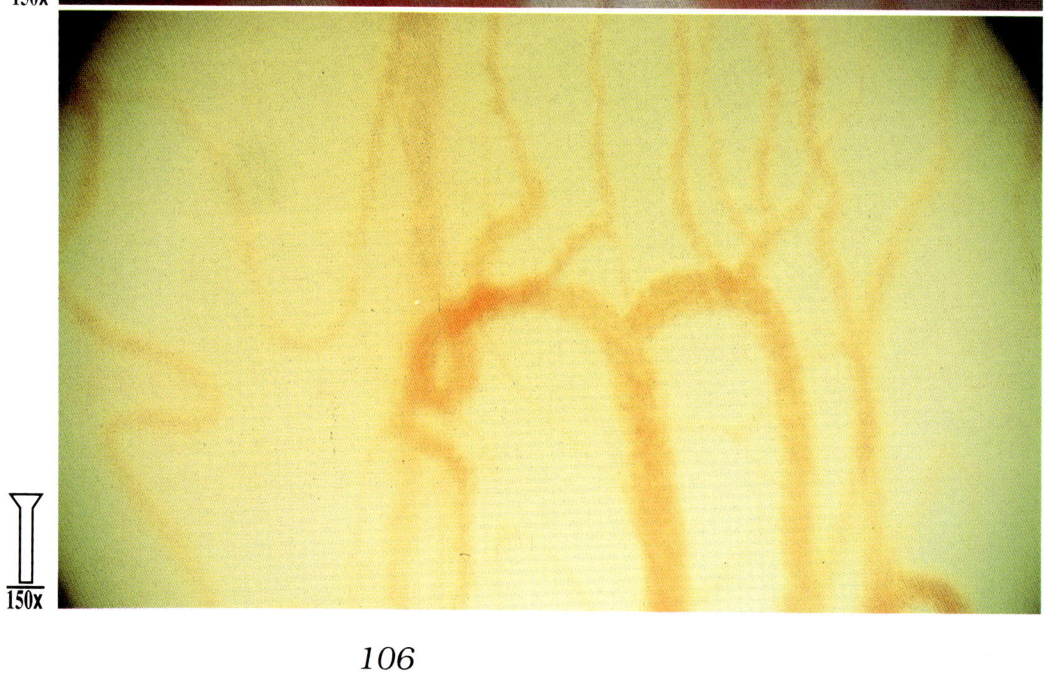
150x

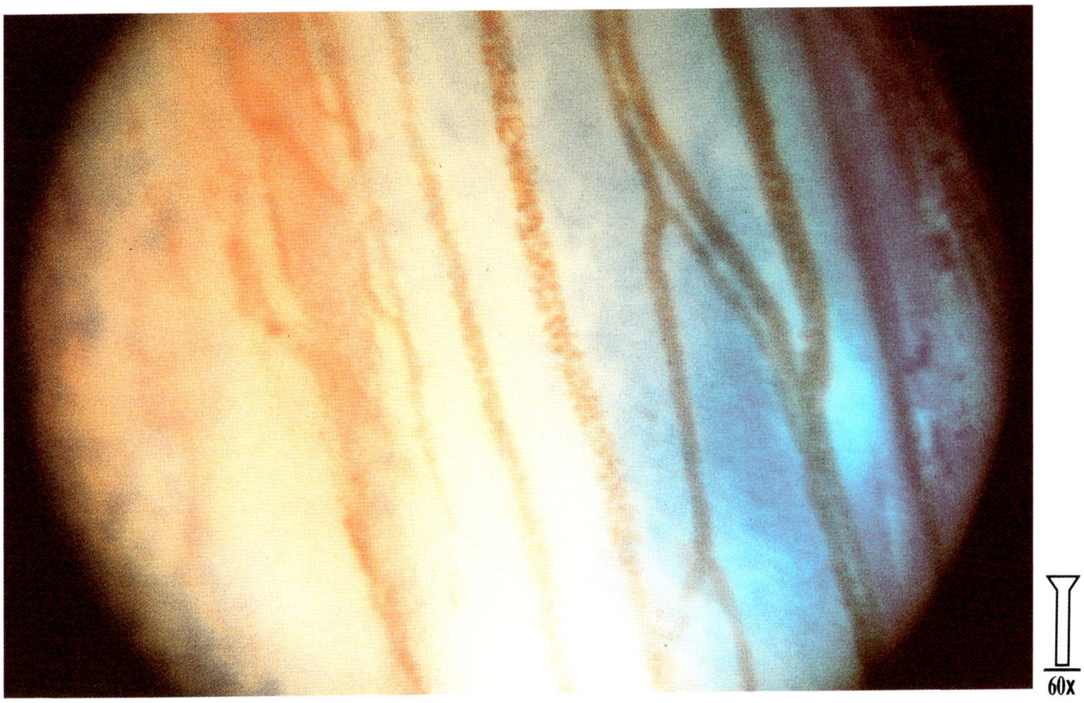

FIG. 97. Normal microvasculature of the vocal cord observed by contact endoscopy (60×).

FIG. 96. Normal microvasculature of the vocal cord observed by contact endoscopy (×150) without methylene blue staining.

60x

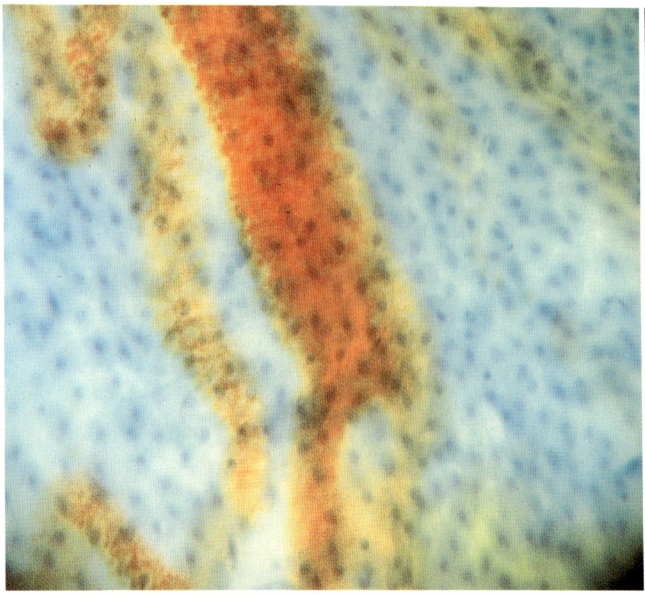

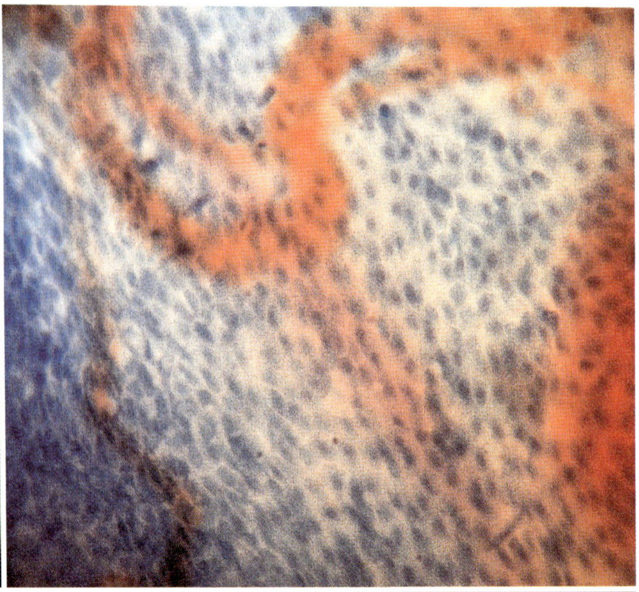

60x

60x

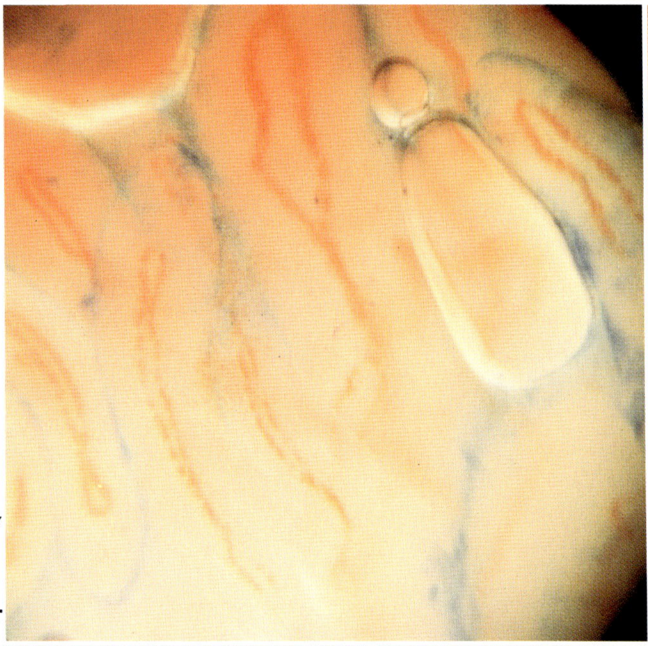

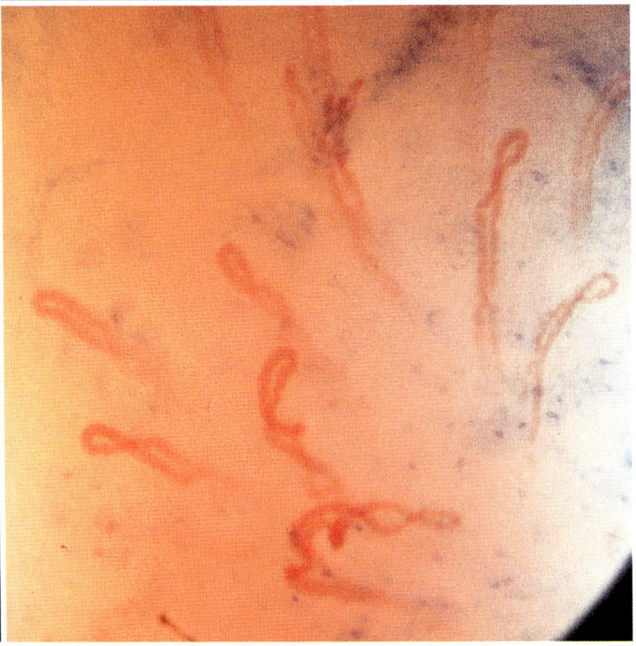

60x

60x

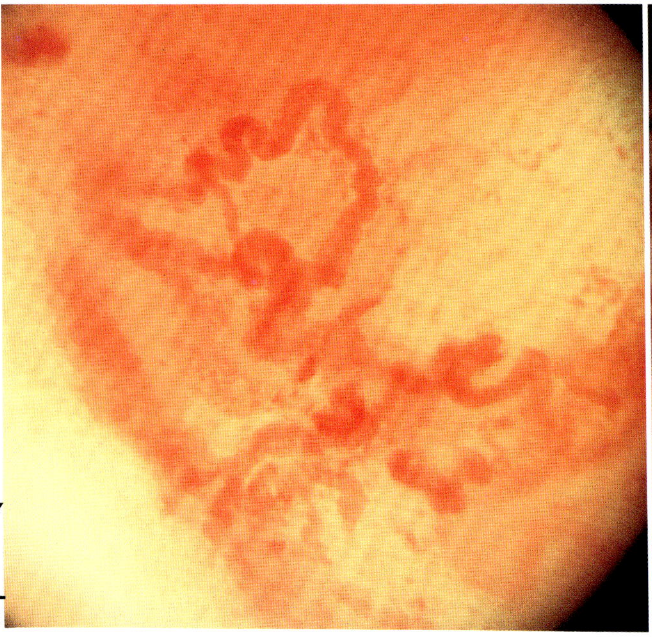

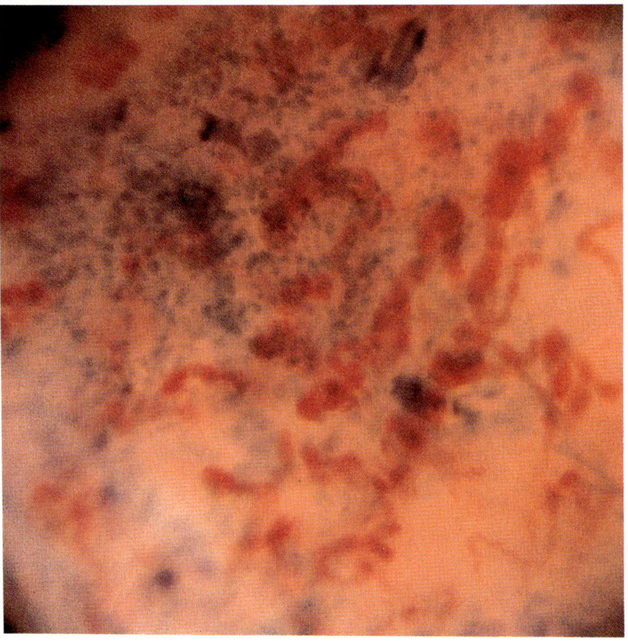

60x

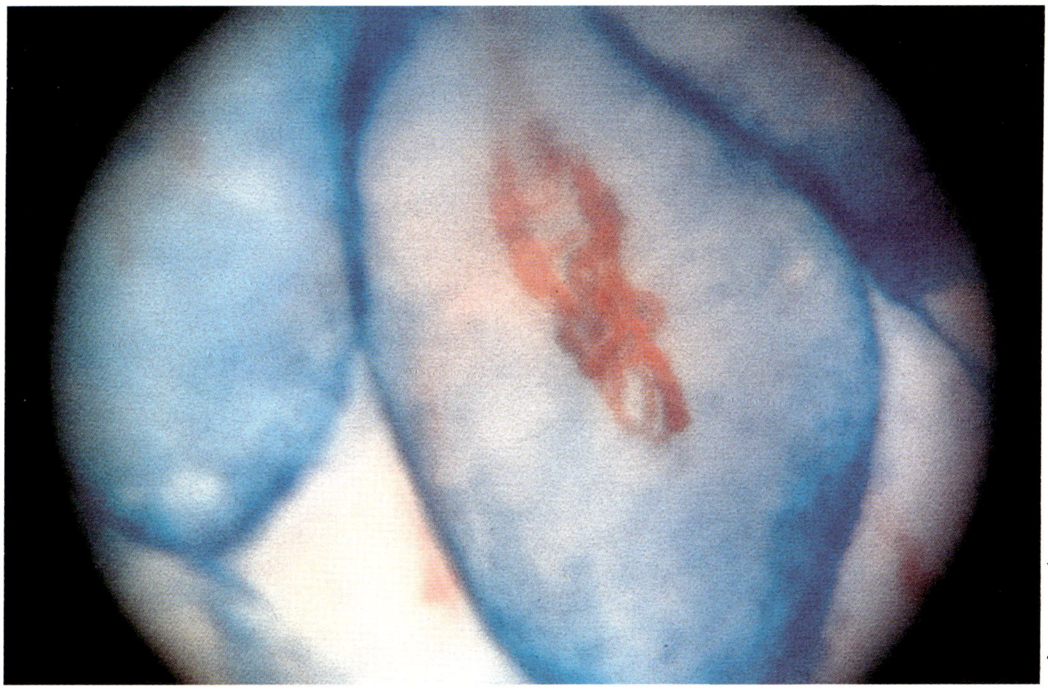

FIG. 99. Contact endoscopy (60×) of a vocal cord papilloma, in which a vascular loop can be identified in the core.

FIG. 98. Blood vessels of the vocal cord observed by contact endoscopy; **A.** Chronic laryngitis; **B.** Chronic laryngitis and keratosis; **C, D.** Papilloma; **E.** Malignant tumor; **F.**

The possibility to see *in vivo* and *in situ* cellular modifications in different diseases, even limited to the superficial layers of the mucosa, is undoubtedly a challenging clinical research project.

The diagnostic features based on histologic sections value the alterations located at the basal layers of the vocal cord epithelium. Contact video endoscopy is not a substitute for biopsies—it is a different evaluation of the tissues in normal and pathological conditions.

With the endoscope (60x and 150x) in contact with the mucosa and following the axis of the vocal cord in all forms of pathology, it is possible to assess the normal and pathological areas and to analyze the transition areas. This allows for a different kind of evaluation of the physiopathology of diseases.

The aim is not to try to observe at the surface what is expected to be seen with classic histologic sections. The goal is to value *in vivo* and *in situ* modifications that occur at the superficial layers, in all of the mucosal surface.

We are still in the first stages of contact endoscopy development—trying to assess its value in biopsy guidance and establishment of safety margins.

Besides all the progress in different areas and technologies that will perfect contact video endoscopy, it is necessary to reinforce the collaboration between clinicians and pathologists.

Almost 15 years have passed since Hamou has brillantly described and developed microcolpohysteroscopy. His work is a landmark.

The clinical applications of contact video endoscopy will progress when other territories and specialities adopt the principles of this technique.

5

References

1. Andrea M. *Vascularização arterial da laringe, distribuição macro e micro vascular* [Ph.D. thesis]. Lisbon, Portugal: University of Lisbon, 1975.
2. Andrea M, Paço J, Guerrier Y. L'Epiglotte et ses amarrages. In: *Cahiers d'ORL et de Chirurgie Cervico-Faciale, XIV.* 1979;8:793–803.
3. Andrea M, Guerrier Y. The anterior commissure of the larynx. *Clin Otolaryngol* 1981;6:259–264.
4. Andrea M. Vasculature of the anterior commissure. *Ann Otol Rhinol Laryngol* 1981;90(1):18–20.
5. Andrea M. Arytenoidectomy. In: *Proceedings of the Workshop and Seminar on Laryngeal Disorders*. Baltimore: Johns Hopkins University, 1992.
6. Andrea M, Paço J, Dias O. The vasculature of the vocal cord. In: *Proceedings of the Collegium ORLAS Meeting*. Cairo, Egypt, 1992.
7. Andrea M, Dias O, Paço J, Santos A. Endoscopia rigida associada a microcirurgia endolaringea, contribuição para o estudo da patologia benigna, pré-maligna e maligna das cordas vocais. *Jornal da Sociedade das Ciências Médicas de Lisboa* (in press).
8. Andrea M, Dias O, Paço J, Santos A. Vocal cord assessment. Rigid and contact endoscopy associated to microlaryngeal surgery. In: *Laryngeal Cancer, Proceedings of the II World Congress on Laryngeal Cancer*. Sydney, Australia: Elsevier Science, 1994.
9. Andrea M, Dias O, Paço J. Endoscopic anatomy of the larynx. *Curr Opin Otol Head Neck Surg* 1994;2:271–275.
10. Andrea M, Dias O, Santos A. Contact endoscopy during microlaryngeal surgery. A new technique for endoscopic examination of the larynx. *Ann Otol Rhinol Laryngol* 1995;104:333–339.
11. Andrea M, Dias O, Santos A. Contact endoscopy of the vocal cord. Normal and pathological patterns. *Acta Otolaryngol (Stockh)* 1995;115:314–316.
12. Andrea M, Dias O. Rigid and contact endoscopy of the larynx. *Arquivos Portugueses de ORL e de Patologia Cervico-Facial* 1994, Suplem. 1, Vol.VIII.
13. Andrea M, Dias O. Rigid and contact endoscopy associated to microlaryngeal surgery. In: Fried M, ed. *The larynx: a multidisciplinary approach (2nd ed)*. Mosby-Year Book (in press).
14. Andrea M, Dias O. La endoscopia rigida e de contacto asociada a la microcirugia laringea. In: *Ponencia de la Sociedad Española de ORL y Patologia Cervico-Facial* (in press).
15. Batsakis J. In: Johnson J.T., Didolkar, M.S. *Head and Neck Cancer*, Vol III. Amsterdam: Elsevier Science 1993;191–196.
16. Benjamin B. *Atlas of paediatric endoscopy of the upper respiratory tract and oesophagus*. New York: Oxford University Press; 1981.
17. Benjamin B. *Diagnostic laryngology: adults and children*. Philadelphia: WB Saunders; 1990.
18. Benjamin B. Prolonged intubation injuries of the larynx: endoscopic diagnosis, classification and treatment. *Ann Otol Rhinol Laryngol* 1993(suppl);160:1–15.
19. Crissman J. Pathology of the upper aerodigestive tract mucosa. In: Paparella M.M, Shumrick D.A., Gluckman J.L., Meyerhoff W.L., eds. *Otolaryngology, Vol. III. Head and Neck, 3rd ed.* Philadelphia: WB Saunders; 1991.
20. Ferlito A. *Neoplasms of the larynx*. New York: Churchill Livingstone; 1993.
21. Folkman J. Towards an understanding of angiogenesis. *Perspect Biol Med* 1985;29(1):11–36.
22. Folkman J, Klagsbrun M. Angiogenic factors. *Science* 1987;235:442–447.
23. Friedrich G, Kainz J, Freidl W. Functional structure of the human vocal cord. *Laryngorhinootologie* 1993;72(5):215–224.

24. Guerrier Y, Andrea M. Microvascularization de la muqueuse laryngée et trachéale. Introduction à la physiopathologie des lésions sténosantes. *Ann Otolaryngol (Paris)* 1980;97(6):409–421.
25. Hamou JE. Microendoscopy and contact endoscopy. Brevet français 79, 04168 Paris, 1979. International patent. PCT/FR 80/0024 Paris 1980. United States patent 4, 385, 810. Washington, 1993.
26. Hamou JE. *Hysteroscopy and microcolpohysteroscopy. Text and atlas* Norwalk, CT; Appleton and Lange: 1991.
27. Hirano M. Phonosurgical anatomy of the larynx. In: Ford C, Bless D, eds. *Phonosurgery: assessment and surgical management of voice disorders*. New York: Raven Press; 1991:25–41.
28. Kantor EA, Berci G, Partlow E, Paz-Partlow H. A completely new approach in microlaryngeal surgery. *Laryngoscope* 1991;101:676–679.
29. Kleinsasser O., Thieme-Verleg G., Kleimsaber O. *Tumors of the larynx and hypopharynx*. Stuttgart, Germany; 1988;349.
30. Kleinsasser O. *Microlaryngoscopy and endolaryngeal microsurgery. 3rd ed.* Philadelphia: Hanley & Belfus, Mosby Year Book; 1991.
31. Lehmann W, Pidoux J, Widmann J. Larynx microlaryngoscopie and histopathologie. Cadempino, Switzerland: Inpharzam Medical; 1981.
32. Maciag T. Cellullar mechanisms of angiogenesis. de Vita V, Hellman S, Rosenberg S, eds. *Important advances in oncology*. Philadelphia: JB Lippincott; 1990:85–98.
33. Martensson B, Fluur E, Schiratzki H. Transconioscopy. A new method of laryngeal investigation. *Acta Otolaryngol (Stockh)* 1964;58:281–284.
34. McGee J. *Oxford textbook of pathology*. New York: Oxford University Press; 1992.
35. Nakaaki K, Shin T. A three dimensional reconstructive study of the layer structure of the human vocal cord. *Eur Arch Otorhinolaryngol* 1993;250(3):190–192.
36. Olofsson J. Histologic grading of early lesions. In: Wigand E, Steiner W, Stell P, eds. *Functional partial laryngectomy*. New York: Springer Verlag; 1984:37–38.
37. Richtsmeier WJ. Head and neck cancer. *Otolaryngol Head Neck Surg* 1992;106:22.
38. Strutz J. 3D endoscopy. *HNO* 1993;41(3):128–130.
39. Vancaille T. *Manual of microcolposcopy*. New York: Elsevier; 1988.
40. Vaughan C. Vocal fold exposure in phonosurgery. *J Voice* 1993;7(2):189–194.
41. Weiland L. Histopathology of early laryngeal carcinoma. In: Wigand E, Steiner W, Stell P, eds. *Functional partial laryngectomy*. New York: Springer Verlag; 1984:31–36.
42. Wheater P, Burkitt H, Daniels V. *Functional histology, 2nd ed.*. New York: Churchill Livingstone; 1991.
43. Yanagisawa E, Yanagisawa R. Laryngeal photography. *Otolaryngol Clin North Am* 1991;24(5):992–1022.
44. Yanagisawa E, Horowitz J, Yanagisawa K, Mambrino L. Comparison of new telescopic video microlaryngoscopic and standard microlaryngoscopic techniques. *Ann Otol Rhinol Laryngol* 1992;101(1):51–60.
45. Yuroto E, Kadota Y, Kurokawa H. Tracheal view of vocal fold vibration in excised canine larynxes. *Arch Otolaryngol Head Neck Surg* 1993;119(1):73–78.

Subject Index